The Institute of Biology's
Studies in Biology no. 53

Bone and
Biomineralization

K. Simkiss
Ph.D.
Professor of Zoology, University of Reading

Edward Arnold

First published 1975
by Edward Arnold (Publishers) Limited
25 Hill Street, London W1X 8LL

Board edition ISBN: 0 7131 2492 X
Paper edition ISBN: 0 7131 2493 8

Printed in Great Britain by
The Camelot Press Ltd, Southampton

General Preface to the Series

It is no longer possible for one textbook to cover the whole field of Biology and to remain sufficiently up-to-date. At the same time teachers and students at school, college or university need to keep abreast of recent trends and know where the most significant developments are taking place.

To meet the need for this progressive approach the Institute of Biology has for some years sponsored this series of booklets dealing with subjects specially selected by a panel of editors. The enthusiastic acceptance of the series by teachers and students at school, college and university shows the usefulness of the books in providing a clear and up-to-date coverage of topics, particularly in areas of research and changing views.

Among features of the series are the attention given to methods, the inclusion of a selected list of books for further reading and, wherever possible, suggestions for practical work.

Reader's comments will be welcomed by the author or the Education Officer of the Institute.

1975

The Institute of Biology,
41 Queens Gate,
London, SW7 5HU

Preface

In this book I have tried to provide some background knowledge to the techniques used by a variety of scientists studying the physiology of bone and other mineralized tissues. I have tried to capture the ideas behind five key experiments together with the methods, results and interpretations necessary to explain them. I am aware that many scientists are considered to live in ivory towers with mistresses of pure truth but, in actual fact, the everyday experiences of many are more akin to sharing a flat with James Thurber. Thus the delights and surprises revealed in these experiments are mainly those of the original researchers and I have tried to avoid the advantages of hindsight in modifying them. For this reason there are some slight historical contradictions between chapters.

It is largely coincidence that each chapter involves a different type of interdisciplinary approach but I hope that this stimulates those who wonder about the need for a broad scientific training. I also hope that those who wonder what contributions an 'observational' biologist has in this scheme will manage to reach the end of the book.

I trust that the book will be accepted on the terms in which it was written: as an honest attempt to avoid a text-book approach. I can see that the approach may annoy some who would prefer to see less experimental detail and discussion and I have therefore attempted to overcome this by summarizing the present state of our knowledge of bone physiology in the final chapter.

Reading,   K. S.
1975

Contents

1 Properties of Calcified Tissues

This book is mainly concerned with five experiments which I have enjoyed reading and thinking about. To my mind they represent fundamental or interesting attempts to discover some of the properties of calcifying tissues. Bone is the best studied example of such a tissue but in order to appreciate it fully, one needs to know a little about the phenomenon of mineralization in general, so that the particular problems of bone physiology can be seen in their true context.

1.1 Biomineralization

The first thing to recognize is that calcium deposits are found in a large number of plants and animals. They occur mainly as carbonates or phosphates, although other compounds such as oxalates and citrates are not uncommon. The most familiar calcified structures are bones, teeth, fish scales, eggshells, snail shells, corals and the spines and tests of a variety of other animals (Table 1–1). It is worth remembering, however, that most of the deposits in the White Cliffs of Dover are actually the products of photosynthesizing coccolithophorids, while the complex

Table 1–1 Types of calcified structures in plants and animals. (PAUTARD, F. G. E. (1966) in *Calcified Tissues*, 1965, Springer, Berlin.)

Group	Carbonates	Phosphates	Oxalates
Invertebrates	Common in most groups as shells, spines, tests, exo and endoskeletons and as statocysts	Present in Protozoa, coelenterates, anthropods and brachiopods	Occasionally in insect eggs and larval cuticles
Vertebrates	In bird and reptile eggshells and otoliths	Bone, dentine and enamel	Found in some soft tissues
Lower plants (Thallophyta, Bryophyta and Pteridophyta)	In cell inclusions	In some bacteria	In some algae, most mosses and ferns
Seed plants (Gymnosperms and Angiosperms)	In cell inclusions	In heartwood	Found in most species

ecosystem of a coral reef is based mainly upon the deposits of algae rather than of animals. Similarly, the oldest evidence for life on earth is probably the 'algal limestones' of Rhodesia which are dated as 2.7×10^9 years old. It appears, therefore, that the ability to form mineralized deposits is a very common property of living systems and if this is accepted then the second point to be considered is why it usually involves calcium rather than some other element.

Calcium is a very common element, weighing about 4 per cent of the earth's crust and this is no doubt one of the reasons it occurs so frequently in animal skeletons. In addition, however, it possesses a relatively large atom which tends to lose its two outer electrons and form the divalent calcium ion. Calcium ions carry a double positive charge but otherwise they have an electron structure like that of the inert gas argon. They tend, therefore, not to share their inner electrons nor to form strong covalent bonds and this is probably why they do not poison many enzymes. Calcium ions have a strong attraction for electrons in oxygen-containing anions such as carbonates, phosphates and sulphates and since these anions are large their outer electrons can also easily break away and become associated with the calcium ion. This reduces the attraction of water for the ions so that these minerals tend to be insoluble. Thus, calcium has three of the most important properties for a skeleton, namely, it is readily available in large quantities, it is non-poisonous and it forms insoluble compounds. Carbonates and phosphates share many of these properties and the body tends to accumulate both of these ions since they form the main inorganic buffers controlling the acidity or pH of an animal. Both ions are also involved in many biochemical reactions so that it is not surprising, in view of their availability, that they are incorporated into shells and skeletons. In fact, as we will see later, it is quite likely that one of the main functions of skeletons is that they can act as stores for these important ions, which can then be released and used again by the body at a later time.

The insolubility of skeletons and shells is one of their obvious properties of great functional significance and the mineral salts involved help to provide the strength, stability and protection which are associated with these structural materials. Mineral salts usually exist in crystalline forms and the majority of skeletons are of this type, although there is now a good deal of evidence to suggest that newly formed bone may contain up to 50 per cent of its minerals in an amorphous state. The exact meaning and significance of this observation is not clear. It may simply be that the crystals are so small that they are not detected by the usual instruments, or it may have some more fundamental explanation (p. 25). For the moment, however, we will consider the minerals of skeletons and shells to exist mainly in a crystalline form, since this provides a valuable insight into many of their properties.

1.2 Crystals

Crystals are characterized by having flat surfaces or faces and by having a certain geometrical regularity or symmetry. This has always been interpreted as indicating that they have a regular and repeating internal structure and the development of X-ray diffraction has now confirmed that this is the case. It is, therefore, possible to talk of a crystal lattice which represents a three-dimensional arrangement of atoms in space. The arrangement of these atoms and the distances between them are fixed for any particular crystal lattice so that it is possible to describe a unit cell as the smallest complete group of these atoms. Crystals can be thought of as being built up by the regular repetition of these polyhedral cells although their structure is, of course, really continuous (Fig. 1–1). A perfect crystal would be one where the arrangement of the atoms fits into a perfect space lattice. In practice it is doubtful whether perfect crystals ever exist, and certainly in biological systems there are always stray impurities which get included in crystals, disrupt the crystal lattice and cause dislocations. These irregularities are of great importance in the growth of crystals. It is often difficult to obtain an increase in the size of a perfect crystal, since the only site for further growth is a two-dimensional surface which has relatively weak interatomic attractions. An imperfect crystal will often contain impurities which disrupt the lattice and produce phenomena such as screw dislocations (Fig. 1–2a). These irregularities can continue to grow by the addition of new atoms into the lattice without it having to start a completely new surface. In these situations growth proceeds in a spiral fashion and numerous examples of these types of crystals appear to be present in animal shells. A similar type of growth occurs when a crystal extends along a single axis which then branches repeatedly. This is called dendritic growth (Fig. 1–2b) and it is also common in shells. Both types of growth continue until they eventually form a single large crystal. Other types of crystal growth are known, but these two types will serve

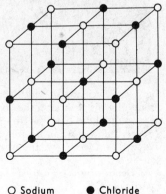

Fig. 1–1 The unit cell of a crystal of sodium chloride showing the regular arrangement of atoms.

○ Sodium   ● Chloride

(a)

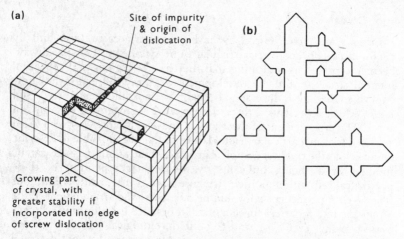

Site of impurity & origin of dislocation

(b)

Growing part of crystal, with greater stability if incorporated into edge of screw dislocation

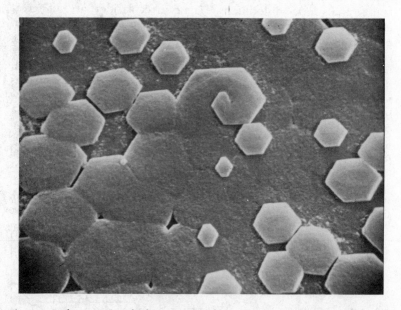

Fig. 1–2 The ways in which some crystals grow. (a) A sequence showing the origin of a dislocation in the crystal lattice at the site of an impurity. A screw dislocation of this type leads to spiral growth of the exposed face. An example of a screw dislocation can be seen in an electron micrograph of the shell of the oyster. (From WISE, S. W. and DE VILLIERS, J. (1971), *Trans. Amer. micros. Soc.,* **90**, 376–80.)

(b) Dendritic growth caused by the extension and branching of a crystal along a particular axis.

to indicate the types of phenomena involved in biological mineralization. The situation in bone is more complex. Bone minerals are rather variable but they have the general formula $Ca_{10}(PO_4)_6(OH)_2$ and are classified as hydroxyapatites. The word 'apatite' comes from the Greek word meaning 'to deceive' and refers to the many problems which mineralogists have had in determining the exact crystallography of these salts. Bone physiologists have experienced the same problems which have been complicated by the fact that individual bone crystals are extremely small, being only about 5 nm (50 Å) in thickness and therefore not capable of being resolved in the light microscope. The small size of the bone crystal means that it has an extremely large surface area compared with its mass and since we have already seen that various ions may attach to crystal surfaces this goes a long way to explain why the overall chemical composition of bone is so variable.

Mineralized skeletons, which are composed of crystals, also possess one other common property and that is that they tend to be bound together with an organic material. This is typically a protein of which collagen is the commonest type and it is usually closely associated with some acidic polysaccharide material. It has been suggested that these organic matrices may play a part in forming the skeleton, but in addition they have important physical properties. Skeletal materials have been compared with 'composites' such as fibreglass where the two components (glass and resin) have different properties from the composite. Certainly bone has a modulus of elasticity intermediate between that of its mineral and organic constituents and a tensile strength greater than either individually. The association between the organic and the mineral parts of most skeletons is extremely intimate and in many cases the protein seems to be integrated into the crystalline structure.

1.3   Biological properties

These then are the basic materials of calcified tissues and so far we have discussed them as if they were mainly physio-chemical phenomena. It is as well to remember, therefore, that they have many other properties of interest to the biologist. Some of these are dealt with in later chapters, but there could not be any better introduction to the significance of skeletons to biologists than by recalling one of the brilliant exercises conducted by the famous anatomist Sir Richard Owen (1803–93).

One day in 1839 Owen was approached by a 'sea-faring man' holding a piece of bone about 6 in. (15 cm) long. The bone had a strong resemblance to the marrow bone of an ox, but the man claimed it was from a giant eagle in New Zealand. After examining it for some time Owen decided that it must be a femur bone from a flightless bird, even larger and heavier than the ostrich. On the basis of this single fragment of bone he was able to give a description of the animal. This was greeted with incredulity and scepticism, since a number of eminent naturalists had by that time visited New Zealand and seen no evidence of such an animal. Thus, when Owen eventually managed to get his observations on the bone published in the Transactions of the Zoological Society, it was with a note that 'the responsibility of the paper rested exclusively with the author'. Owen, however, named the bird *Dinornis struthioides* ('huge bird like an Ostrich') and sent a number of reprints of his article to colleagues in New Zealand. Four years later he received from them a collection of bones from which he was able to reconstruct a whole skeleton of the extinct Moa which completely substantiated his predictions (Fig. 1–3).

This example of scientific deduction and detective work was based on two main principles. One was the anatomical concept of homology which Owen introduced and defined as 'The same organ in different animals under every variety of form and function' and which is now interpreted as indicating genetic relationships between animals. By this means Owen was able to make extensive deductions about the other bones which would have been associated with a femur. The other basic principle which allowed him to deduce so much from a single bone was the fact that it was adapted to withstand the stresses put upon it during life. Thus the lumps and ridges found on bones enable a skilled anatomist to deduce what muscles were attached and how the weight was distributed about the bone. Bones in fact appear to be capable of being treated as if they had, during life, shown structural responses to the engineering problems of the support and movement of the animal.

The two principles utilized by Owen remain as basic concepts in skeletal anatomy, but relatively little has been added to many aspects of our knowledge of skeletal physiology. This is very surprising since most skeletons appear to consist of a relatively simple deposit of inorganic salts around cells and one might reasonably expect this to be an easy system to investigate. Certainly when compared with the complexities of most of the organs of the body, which involve such diverse biochemical syntheses and complex intracellular activities, the skeleton seems to be a relatively uncomplicated if somewhat neglected organ. One final comment is, however, of interest. The adaptive aspects of bone formation are one of the most interesting properties of skeletons, but it is not just bones which modify themselves according to the stresses placed upon them. Nearly all the organs and tissues of the body—eyes, brains, lungs, kidneys, blood vessels, testes, etc.—are capable of developing mineralized deposits. These deposits appear frequently in organs after infections, during ageing or at the time of wound healing and it has been claimed, for example, that after excessive riding cavalrymen have developed such ectopic bone in their buttocks. The

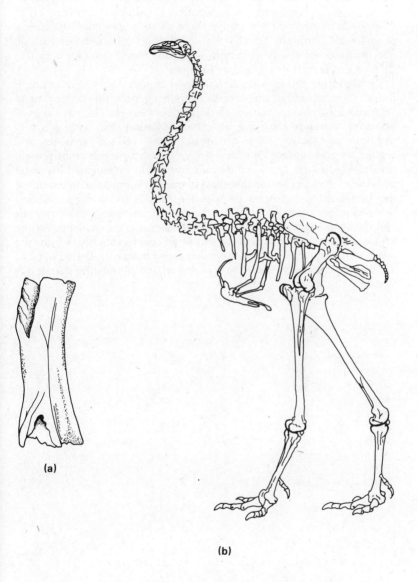

(a)

(b)

Fig. 1–3   (a) The fragment of bone presented to Sir Richard Owen and (b) the complete skeleton of a Moa reconstructed later. (Redrawn from *The Life of Richard Owen* by R. OWEN (1894) and *Fossil Birds* by W. E. SWINTON (1958), British Museum.)

whole phenomenon of extra skeletal mineralization is considered by Hans Selye to represent a fundamental biological process called calciphylaxis. According to Selye there exists a 'regulated biological mechanism through which the organism can induce calcium precipitation selectively at certain sites and thereby initiate localized defensive inflammatory responses to injury'.

Perhaps from this introduction it might appear that mineralization is indeed a very simple phenomenon requiring only the deposition of relatively insoluble crystals on an organic framework. This viewpoint is, however, currently changing with the realization that bone is a very dynamic and active tissue involving many cellular activities and regulatory phenomena. Our knowledge of these aspects is at the present time rather limited, but when they are more fully investigated it may be possible to see whether the skeletal system is the ultimate achievement of the mineralization process or whether the ability to form calcified deposits is an important aspect of the general physiology of all animals and tissues as suggested by Selye. That, however, is the challenge for the future and the experiments in the following chapters simply indicate the way that our current concepts have developed from considering bone as an inert supporting structure to realizing what a stimulating system it is to study.

2   The Solubility of Skeletons

We have already seen that calcified skeletons have two important properties. The first is that they consist of a large collection of relatively insoluble crystals which are deposited from the body fluids in certain specialized parts of the animal. The second is that this crystallization normally occurs on an organic base or matrix which becomes incorporated into the material of the skeleton.

The first experiment we will consider arose directly from these two properties. In effect it attempted to apply to biological systems the simple chemical laws which govern the solubilities of crystals.

Crystals dissolve in water because the outermost ions in the crystal lattice have a tendency to break away from the surface and become detached. The presence of water actually facilitates this process and if many ions become separated from the crystal we say that it has dissolved in the water, whereas if only a few ions pass into solution we say the crystal is rather insoluble. It is important to realize, however, that there is no basic distinction between these two types of crystal.

If a sufficiently large piece of a crystal is put into water the ions will continue to dissolve and produce a progressively more concentrated solution. As this process continues it increases the probability that some of the ions dissolved in the water will bump into each other or into the original crystal, and thus produce some more solid mineral. Thus an equilibrium point will eventually be reached at which the tendency for an ion to pass into solution is exactly matched by the tendency for the ions in solution to bump into the crystal and come out of solution again (Fig. 2–1). When this occurs the solution is said to be saturated for that particular salt.

The law which summarizes the conditions for saturation simply states that the product of the concentration of the ions in solution is always a constant under any given set of conditions. Thus for a calcareous shell in sea water the 'solubility product constant' at 30°C is 1.62×10^{-6} $(mol/l)^2$. Normally under these conditions sea water contains 10^{-2} mol/l calcium and 1.62×10^{-4} mol/l carbonate ions and it is therefore saturated with calcium carbonate, i.e.

$$(10^{-2}) \times (1.62 \times 10^{-4}) \doteqdot 1.62 \times 10^{-6}$$
$$[Ca^{2+}] \qquad [CO_3^{2-}] \qquad CaCO_3$$

If we take a solution containing many different kinds of ions the solubility product constant becomes more complex since all the ions in solution tend to interfere with each other's movements and reduce the

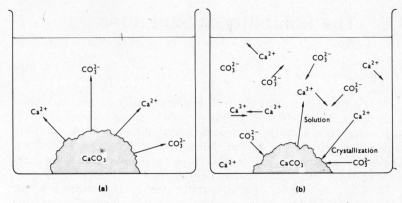

Fig. 2–1 The solubility of calcium carbonate in distilled water. (a) Calcium and carbonate ions break away from the surface of the crystal and pass into solution. (b) As more and more of the crystal dissolves the solution becomes more concentrated. The ions in solution will then collide with each other and with the crystal to reform solid. When the process of ion loss predominates the crystal dissolves. When the collision process predominates precipitation or crystallization occurs. When the two processes are in equilibrium the solution is saturated.

number of effective collisions. The solubility product constant considered above was for sea water containing 36 g of salt in 1000 g of sea water and less calcium carbonate would dissolve in diluted sea water. Temperature similarly affects the movement of ions in solution and thus their solubility product constant.

The reason for discussing the solubility of crystals is, I hope, now clear. The mineralization of biological tissues will only occur if the fluid at the site of calcification contains so many of the constituent ions that they exceed the solubility product constant.

The experiment we will now follow attempted to discover whether the blood and extracellular fluids of a mammal were saturated with bone minerals or not. The results were very surprising, but before considering them we should note the care with which the experiments were carried out.

2.1   The experiments

This work was undertaken by W. F. NEUMAN and H. FLEISCH and published in a number of articles in 1960.

In these experiments a large number of flasks were carefully cleaned and salt solutions were prepared by dissolving pure chemicals in boiled distilled water. The pH of the solutions was buffered at 7.4 by using dimethyl barbituric acid free of contaminating ions. The total number of ions in each solution was kept constant by adjusting the final concentration with potassium chloride (KCl). Salts were always dissolved in the same order, i.e. potassium dihydrogen phosphate (KH_2PO_4), barbitone buffer, potassium chloride (KCl) and then calcium chloride ($CaCl_2$). The calcium concentration was kept constant at 1.67 mmol/l, but the quantity of phosphorus present as inorganic phosphate (P_i) was altered so that the product of $Ca \times P_i$ varied eightfold from 0.83 to 6.67 $(mmol/l)^2$ covering conditions of undersaturation to supersaturation. Chloroform or the antibiotic *neomycin* was also added to prevent bacterial growth. The solutions were sealed in an atmosphere of nitrogen by means of a layer of paraffin wax over the top of the flasks. In some cases small amounts of defatted and ground up bone mineral were added to the flasks. In other cases the protein collagen was obtained from various sites (calf skin, tendon, etc.) and purified by dissolving it in 0.45 mol/l sodium chloride from which it was reprecipitated and then added to the flasks of salt solutions. The flasks were kept at a constant temperature and shaken for three days. They were then opened, the pH measured and the solutions analysed for their calcium and phosphate content. Any minerals formed in the flasks were also analysed.

Solutions which originally contained very small amounts of phosphate at the start of the experiment but which had had small samples of bone mineral added to them before incubation were shown on analysis to give a $Ca \times P_i$ product of 0.8 $(mmol/l)^2$. Other solutions without mineral showed no difference from the $Ca \times P_i$ that was originally placed in the flask until products of 2.5 to 4.3 $(mmol/l)^2$ were reached. The precipitation of mineral similar in composition to bone did not occur until $Ca \times P_i$ products of over 4.3 $(mmol/l)^2$ were obtained. The presence of calf skin collagen did not influence this, but solutions containing collagen from tendons never contained $Ca \times P_i$ products of more than 1.3 $(mmol/l)^2$. Some of these results are shown in Table 2–1. The column labelled 'Standard deviation of the mean' is a statistical measure of how much variation occurs in the results when the same experiments are repeated several times.

2.2 Discussion and results

Essentially these were very simple experiments, but they are noteworthy for the great care that was taken in their execution. Thus, the distilled water was always boiled and the samples were kept under nitrogen so that all carbon dioxide was excluded. Carbon dioxide in solution might form carbonic acid and upset the experiment by precipitating calcium carbonate. The salts to be used were always dissolved in the same order so as to minimize the chance of precipitating small deposits during the preparation of the solutions. Bacteria were also excluded, since these might add or remove ions from solution and thus upset the apparent solubility products. The temperature was kept constant, the pH was constant and the total concentration of ions in the solution was constant. This was necessary, since all these factors affect the solubilities of salts. The flasks were also shaken for the same period of time in every case. If many factors vary it is very difficult to repeat an experiment or interpret the results. The success of these precautions can be seen in the results shown in Table 2–1. The standard deviation of the mean is very small, i.e. statistical tests indicate that the results are very reproducible. Normally 95 per cent of all results fall within two standard deviations of the mean. Thus, if the experiment of finding the solubility product of $Ca \times P_1$ shown in Table 2–1 was repeated 100 times then in 95 cases the results would be in the range of $4.30-(2 \times 0.016)$ to $4.30+(2 \times 0.016)$, i.e. a range of 4.27 to 4.33 with a mean of 4.30.

Table 2–1   The $Ca \times P_1$ values of solutions 3 days after being made up at initial values of 4.3 $(mmol/l)^2$. (Data recalculated after FLEISH, H. and NEUMAN, W. F. (1961), *Am. J. Physiol.* **200**, 1296–1300.)

State of solution	Number of Experiments	$Ca \times P_1 \ (mmol/l)^2$	Standard deviation of mean
Contains no collagen	7	4.30	± 0.016
Contains calf skin collagen	5	2.50–4.30	—
Contains tendon collagen	9	1.30	± 0.046

Another important fact also emerges from these experiments. The experimenters have tried to see if adding pieces of the protein collagen affects the solubility products they are investigating. They have realized, however, that collagen is a term used for a large group of proteins which differ slightly in their composition and purity. They have, therefore, tried to purify the protein before using it and have always noted what type of collagen they used. This is most important since the results obtained using calf skin collagen are very different from those with tendon collagen (Table 2–1).

All of these precautions ensure that the experimental data are reliable and repeatable. Only then can one be absolutely sure that the results have not been caused by stray influences in the work. The importance of all this care is apparent when the results are unexpected as in this experiment. It means that the scientist can now try and explain the mechanism responsible for his data rather than worry about whether inaccuracies or errors caused the results.

The plasma of the blood of mammals contains about 1.67 mmol/l of ionic calcium and about 1.0 mmol/l inorganic phosphorus. This gives a $Ca \times P_1$ value of about 1.67 $(mmol/l)^2$. Bone mineral dissolves to give a

$Ca \times P_1$ solubility product constant of about 0.83 $(mmol/l)^2$. It would appear on this basis that the blood is supersaturated with bone mineral which should therefore crystallize out of solution all over the body. But artificial solutions similar in composition to plasma do not cause minerals to precipitate out of solution until the abnormally high $Ca \times P_1$ values of about 4.3 $(mmol/l)^2$ are obtained. On this basis the blood is normally undersaturated for bone mineral. These facts are summarized in Fig. 2–2, which highlights the strange anomaly demonstrated by these experiments. It is a paradox that when one tries to dissolve bone minerals in an artificial blood the solution appears to be supersaturated, but when one tries to precipitate bone out of it it behaves as if it was undersaturated. At first sight this is ridiculous, for there should only be one solubility product constant for bone mineral, whether one approaches it from supersaturation or undersaturation.

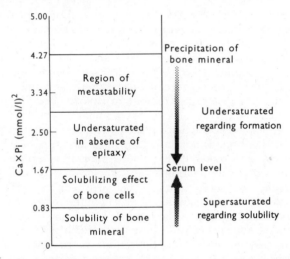

Fig. 2–2   The calcium and phosphate products necessary to precipitate bone mineral (apatite) in relation to the level of ions in the blood and the solubility of bone mineral. Note that the blood is apparently supersaturated with regard to the solubility of bone mineral. (Recalculated using data from FLEISCH, H. and NEUMAN, W. F. (1960), *J. Amer. Chem. Soc.*, **82**, 996–7.)

2.3   The interpretation

W. F. NEUMAN and his wife MARGARET W. NEUMAN tried to resolve this situation in their book *The Chemical Dynamics of Bone Mineral*. They suggested that the body fluids were indeed supersaturated with bone mineral, so that the major anomaly was in interpreting the difficulty in precipitating bone mineral. The important word here is 'precipitating' for there is a subtle distinction between liquids which are in contact with crystals and those which have to form the crystals from solutions which contain no solid matter. The first aggregations of ions to combine and start to form a crystal are highly unstable, since they have a very large surface area relative to their volume. Such minute crystals very easily redissolve because the surface area available for the escape of ions is large compared with the small number of ions inside the crystal tending to hold them in place. Much higher concentrations of ions are necessary in order to induce new crystal formation when compared with the concentration required for continued crystal growth. It was suggested, therefore, that the very high ionic products of $Ca \times P_l$ found in the experiment simply demonstrated the difficulty in initiating the formation of new crystals. If crystals had already existed in the solution they would have been able to grow and form larger crystals at much smaller ionic concentrations. This concept explained the experimental difficulty of inducing precipitates of bone mineral but it provided little explanation as to how bone mineralization might normally occur in the body. It did, however, provide a clue. It is known that if two different types of crystal have similar distributions and types of ionic charges in their lattice then one type of crystal will grow over the surface of the other. Such occurrences are rare but, for example, ammonium bromide will crystallize on the surface of sodium chloride crystals because in certain directions the two crystals have similar lattice structures (Fig. 2–3). This phenomenon is known as 'epitaxy' or crystal overgrowth. Could it be that bone is normally formed in certain parts of the body because there are structures which allow mineral to form by epitactic growth rather than precipitation?

The exciting suggestion was made that the protein fibre collagen may, in certain circumstances, have along its length the correct arrangement and size of charged groups to be epitactic to a crystal of bone mineral. Bone would then be expected to form on these fibres by crystal growth at calcium and phosphate concentrations much lower than those necessary to precipitate the mineral. Reference to the results in Table 2–1 shows that this does in fact occur. Certain types of collagen will initiate mineralization at ionic products of 1.3 $(mmol/l)^2$, i.e. at slightly lower levels than actually occur in normal blood.

On the basis of these experiments it was suggested that the body fluids are normally supersaturated for bone mineral. Crystals do not form at random in the body, since the energy necessary to initiate the first crystal nuclei is much greater than normally occurs. This barrier to mineralization could, however, be removed if pre-existing mineral was available, or if collagen fibres in the correct form were present. Crystals would then be formed by the process of epitaxy over the protein template, which could be considered as normally only being found at sites of bone formation.

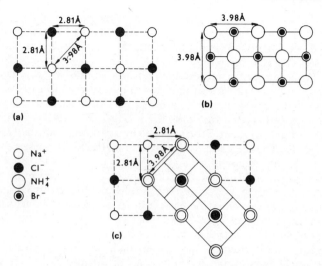

Fig. 2–3 (a) The crystal lattice of sodium chloride showing that adjacent sodium ions are 3.98 Å apart. (b) The crystal lattice of ammonium bromide with a distance of 3.98 Å between ammonium ions. (c) Ammonium bromide growing over the surface of a sodium chloride crystal by epitaxy. The phenomenon of epitaxy occurs because the crystal lattices overlap if placed at 45° to each other. Crystal overgrowth occurs only where it is possible to have a close fit between the two different crystal lattices. (10 Ångstrom = 1 nm)

2.4   Later work

There is now a great deal of accumulated evidence to suggest that collagen fibres play an important part in the calcification of bone. The idea that this might be the case predates Neuman's work by many years, but the work we have discussed had the advantage of also suggesting that two important phenomena may be involved in calcification. The first was that the body fluids were supersaturated with bone mineral, and the second was that minerals only crystallized on certain collagen fibres because these had the correct structure to act as surfaces for crystal growth. Both of these concepts have been applied to other systems on the assumption that they represent fundamental aspects of bio-mineralization.

The suggestion that the body fluids may be supersaturated is rather difficult to investigate. It is certainly true that crystals will neither form nor grow unless the solution surrounding them is continually tending towards supersaturation. The sites of calcification are, however, often somewhat removed from the main volume of the body fluids and it is quite possible that the conditions of supersaturation only exist in the locality of the site of calcification. In addition, there are the analytical complications that much of the calcium in the body fluids is protein bound and not involved in ionic phenomena and the two anions involved, i.e. carbonate and phosphate, also exist in many different forms (HCO_3^-, H_2CO_3, HPO_4^{2-}, $H_2PO_4^-$) which vary with pH. Despite these complications it is interesting to note the work of W. T. W. POTTS, who analysed the blood of various molluscs and attempted to work out the ionic products of calcium and carbonate. These results are shown in Table 2–2 together with the solubility product constant for aragonite, the more soluble of the two forms of calcium carbonate normally found in snail shells. The calculations of POTTS are corrected for protein-bound calcium, for pH, temperature and the effects of salinity and show that the blood of these invertebrates also appears to be supersaturated for the material of their skeletons. The results are suggestive enough to make one wonder whether the basic principles discussed by NEUMAN are also applicable to other animals and other skeletons.

This thought probably also occurred to a number of scientists in the 1960s, for several attempts have been made to see if the protein in mollusc shells is epitactic for the crystals of calcium carbonate which normally occur on it. Mollusc shells are, in fact, particularly interesting in this respect because although they are nearly all composed of calcium carbonate some of them have this in the crystalline form of aragonite, whereas others have it in the less soluble form of calcite. It is, therefore, possible to design an ingenious test for the theory of epitaxy by taking pieces of the protein from the aragonite shells of the freshwater clam *(Elliptio complanatus)* or the pearl oyster *(Pinctada martensii)* and putting them between the shell and the tissues of the oyster *(Crassostrea virginica)*. The oyster, *C. virginica*, normally forms a calcite shell, so that if the inserted protein recalcified as aragonite it would suggest that the introduced organic material had influenced the type of crystal which formed upon it. The experiment was performed in 1960 by N. WATABE and K. M. WILBUR and the results are shown in Table 2–3. Most people would interpret these results as suggestive of epitactic influences, but they are far from being conclusive. Other evidence tends to support the

Table 2–2 The ionic product ($Ca \times CO_3$) of the blood of various molluscs in relation to the solubility product of calcium carbonate (as aragonite). (Data from POTTS, W. T. W. (1954), *J. exp. Biol.* **31**, 376–85.)

Sample	$Ca \times CO_3$ conc. in blood $(mmol/l)^2$	Solubility product of aragonite in similar conditions $(mmol/l)^2$	State
Mytilus blood	2.31×10^{-6}	1.95×10^{-6}	Supersaturated
Anodonta blood	0.33×10^{-6}	0.09×10^{-6}	Supersaturated
Helix blood	0.60×10^{-6}	0.55×10^{-6}	Supersaturated

(a) Eggshell

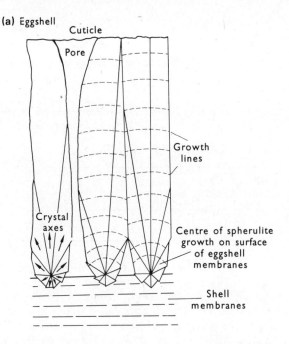

Cuticle

Pore

Growth lines

Crystal axes

Centre of spherulite growth on surface of eggshell membranes

Shell membranes

(b) Japanese oyster shell

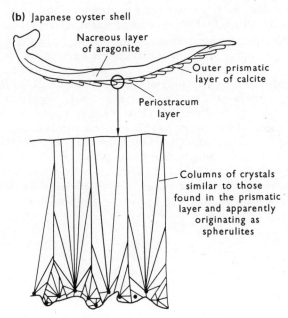

Nacreous layer of aragonite

Outer prismatic layer of calcite

Periostracum layer

Columns of crystals similar to those found in the prismatic layer and apparently originating as spherulites

Fig. 2–4 Radial sections through (a) an avian eggshell and (b) a bivalve mollusc shell, showing centres of spherulite crystal growth. (Partly after TAYLOR, J. D., KENNEDY, W. J. and HALL, A. (1969), *Bull. Brit. Mus. (Nat. Hist.) Zoology* suppl. 3.)

Table 2–3   The influence of the organic matric of aragonite shells of molluscs upon the normal process of calcite deposition in oysters *(Crassostrea virginica)*. (Data from WATABE, N. and WILBUR, K. M. (1960), *Nature, Lond.* **188**, 334.)

Source of protein matrix	Total number of matrix pieces analysed	Number of pieces with aragonite crystals
Japanese pearl oyster *(Pinctada martensii)*	4	2
Freshwater clam *(Elliptio complanatus)*	8	1
Total	12 (100%)	3 (25%)

idea and if, for example, one looks at pieces of birds' eggshells or pieces of certain snail shells (Fig. 2–4) one finds that the crystals which form the shell are initiated by small masses of protein from which crystals grow out in all directions to form what are called spherulites. Are these small masses of protein epitactic for these shell crystals? It is certainly an interesting suggestion, but crystallographers are familiar with the fact that spherulites are notoriously easy to form and thus the support given to the epitaxy theory by these observations is again far from conclusive.

Collagen itself remains, therefore, the best studied protein in relation to possible epitaxy. Electron micrographs have shown that the first crystals of bone which form on the collagen fibres are precisely orientated with their crystallographic *c* axes parallel to the long axis of the fibre (Fig. 2–5). These crystals are closely aligned to the cross striations seen on collagen fibres and it has frequently been suggested that the chemical groups responsible for these particular striations form the epitactic surface on which bone formation occurs. Much of the current work on the composition and structure of collagen is now being pursued with the intention of clarifying this suggestion which is clearly of fundamental importance to our understanding of the phenomenon of biomineralization.

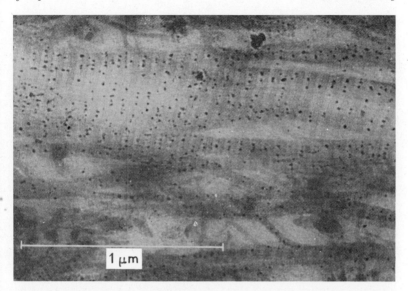

Fig. 2–5   Collagen fibres in the bone of a 16-day-old chick embyro. Note the crossbanding of the collagen and the small mineral particles associated with this repeating unit. (From FITTON-JACKSON, S. (1957), *Proc. R. Soc.*, **146B**, 270–80.)

3 Crystal Poisons

The situations in which scientists get their ideas for new experiments are obviously very varied, but undoubtedly one of the best ways is by comparing their work with that of their colleagues. This may occur by reading about other people's work or by actually discussing it with them. The process is very rarely documented for it is usually some years before the results of an experiment are completed, written up and published and it is then presented in a logical rather than an historical form. An exception to this has occurred in recent years when some scientific conferences have been recorded verbatim so that discussions of experiments are published roughly as they took place. Such a conference was organized in 1950 by the Macy Foundation and published in a series of volumes entitled *Metabolic Interrelations*. The conferences were largely on mineralized tissues and during the consideration of a paper by two biochemists, Gutman and Yu, there was some discussion of the role of certain enzymes in the process of cartilage calcification. In order to appreciate the background to this discussion, however, we have to go back over fifty years.

One of the earliest theories of bone formation was proposed by R. ROBISON. In 1923 he was studying the distribution of the enzyme alkaline phosphatase which catalyses the hydrolysis of phosphate esters, e.g.

glucose phosphate → glucose + inorganic phosphate.

Some of his results are shown in Table 3–1 and the high concentration of the enzyme in the calcifying cartilage of femur bone is very apparent. The observation took on added significance when the results were compared with those obtained from non-calcifying cartilage such as that of rib. Robison, who was a brilliant experimentalist, soon realized that the distribution of the enzyme provided the basis for a theory of

Table 3–1 The quantity of the enzyme alkaline phosphatase in various tissues of the rat. (Data from ROBISON, R. (1923), *Biochem. J.*, **17**, 286–93.)

Tissue	% ester phosphate hydrolysed
Calcifying cartilage (femur epiphyses)	90
Non-calcifying cartilage (rib)	2
Trachea	3
Liver	11
Spleen	7
Heart muscle	9

mineralization, since the enzyme would release inorganic phosphates from the organic phosphates in the blood. This local excess of phosphate ions would tend to exceed the solubility product of bone mineral at the site of the enzyme so that calcification would be induced there.

This theory of bone formation is undoubtedly wrong, but it has persisted in textbooks despite the fact that Robison himself realized that there were only trace amounts (10^{-4} mol/l) of ester phosphates in blood plasma. Furthermore, even these quantities of organic phosphates are poorly hydrolysed by the enzyme alkaline phosphatase. In later years ROBISON relegated this enzyme to a less fundamental role in his scheme of calcification but others have continued to invoke it. In this respect it is important to distinguish clearly between theories and facts. The demonstration that ROBISON's theory is no longer acceptable does not modify the fact that there is usually a very good correlation between sites of calcification and the histological occurrence of the enzyme. For this reason the enzyme alkaline phosphatase has always fascinated bone physiologists.

With that background information we can now appreciate NEUMAN's comments in the following discussion which took place at the conference discussing the role of enzymes in calcification.

HASTINGS: . . . But Dr. Gutman gave me a perfectly wild idea while he was talking there. How about this: ATP (adenosine triphosphate) being a storage of phosphate to prevent calcification until you really want it. . . . We know the calcium is in this . . . part of cartilage. That is a very good source of extra calcium that you cannot account for otherwise. Anyway the calcium is there. You have a bond. Put a pyrophosphate on there and you cannot go any further. You are through.

NEUMAN: *That may be the function of phosphatase: to prevent the accumulation of organic phosphates which would effectively block the surface and prevent crystal growth.*

HASTINGS: That's an answer.

The conference then continued to discuss enzymes in cells. NEUMAN, however, obviously left the discussion with the germ of the idea that perhaps the enzyme phosphatase was important in calcification, not because it started the process (as envisaged by ROBISON), but because it removed an inhibitor that was stopping the process from occurring spontaneously. One can detect in this idea the implications of his previous work on supersaturation (Chapter 2) and W. F. NEUMAN was obviously thinking that calcification should occur spontaneously and worrying more about why this didn't happen, rather than about how it was initiated. NEUMAN therefore set out to try and see if the blood contained inhibitors to calcification and at the next conference on *Metabolic Interrelations* he was able to report considerable success in this work. A complete investigation of the phenomenon was, however, to take more than 10 years to complete and we will therefore consider the later publications of H. FLEISCH and W. F. NEUMAN.

3.1 The experiment

The experiment took place in two parts. First, the demonstration that an inhibitor was present and second, the identification of it chemically.

In order to demonstrate that the blood contained an inhibitor of mineralization FLEISCH and NEUMAN simply modified some of the experiments that we have already considered in the previous chapter. Solutions which contained 1.67 mmol/l calcium were prepared in the same careful way and the inorganic phosphate content was varied to give $Ca \times P_1$ values of from 2.5 to 11.7 (mmol/l)^2. The solutions were shaken in the presence of collagen fibres, known to be capable of inducing mineral formation and after 3 days they were removed and analysed. The procedure was then varied by taking some plasma from the blood of a dog and forcing it under pressure through a semipermeable dialysis membrane. Dialysis membranes of this type only allow the small electrolytes to pass through them so that it is possible to separate the salts from the proteins by simply collecting the ultrafiltrate. This was in fact done and 8 parts of plasma ultrafiltrate were added to 92 parts of the artificial salt solution before repeating the experiment. It was found that the solution containing the plasma extract prevented calcification from occurring. Furthermore, if the plasma was incubated with the enzyme alkaline phosphatase before use the inhibitor was destroyed. The results of these experiments are shown in Table 3–2.

Having demonstrated that the blood appeared to contain an inhibitor of calcification the next problem was to isolate and identify the material

Table 3–2 The minimum ionic products necessary to initiate crystal formation from solutions in the presence of collagen fibres (cf. Table 2–1). Note how dog plasma prevents crystal formation and how this ability is lost on incubating the blood with alkaline phosphatase. (Date recalculated from FLEISCH, H. and NEUMAN, W. F. (1961), *Am. J. Physiol.*, **200**, 1296–1300.)

	Final ionic products required for crystal formation $Ca \times P_1$ (mmol/l)^2	Standard deviation of mean
Control saline	1.33	± 0.04
Diluted dog plasma	2.83	± 0.34
Diluted dog plasma after treatment with alkaline phosphatase	1.91	± 0.22

chemically. But how could they set about such a seemingly endless task? First, FLEISCH and NEUMAN argued that since the material was present in the ultrafilterable part of the blood it should also be present in the urine, since ultrafiltration is the basic mechanism of urine formation by the kidney. Urine is much more readily available than blood and they soon showed that it too inhibited calcification.

It was implicit in the way that NEUMAN developed the idea of the inhibitor that he expected it to be a phosphate-containing substance and the experiment with alkaline phosphatase tended to confirm this (Table 3–2).

In order to isolate the compound they passed large quantities of urine down an ion exchange column. This consists of a glass tube packed with resin beads each of which carries positively charged groups which tend to bind negatively charged anions. Urine which had passed through such a column contained no inhibitor and it was therefore assumed that the inhibitor remained attached to the resin. It was freed from this attachment by passing 0.5 mol/l potassium chloride at pH 8.4 down the ion exchange column. The isolated inhibitor was purified by adding to it 10 volumes of a 3 : 1 mixture of alcohol and ether. It was then precipitated with barium salts and a sample of the precipitate was exposed to X-ray diffraction. This is a common way of identifying crystals since the X-rays are diffracted in a way which is characteristic for each crystal lattice. The pattern of diffraction lines can be recorded on film, measured and then identified by reference to tables of known standards. It was thus possible to identify the crystals as barium pyrophosphate ($Ba_2P_2O_7$) and eventually similar pyrophosphate ions were isolated from the blood at concentrations of less than 10^{-5} mol/l. In these trace amounts they inhibited the formation of bone mineral and apparently stopped normal calcification.

3.2   The interpretation

The demonstration and identification of an inhibitor of calcification is quite convincing. There is, however, a problem in understanding how this inhibition comes about. Thus, the concentrations of the relevant ions in plasma are calcium, 1.67 mmol/l; inorganic phosphates 1.00 mmol/l; pyrophosphate inhibitor 0.01 mmol/l. The inhibitor is present at a concentration many times less than the concentrations of the ions forming bone mineral, so it obviously does not produce its effect by binding on to these ions and destroying them. How then does it act in such small concentrations to inhibit the formation of hydroxyapatite crystals?

One suggestion which has been made is that pyrophosphate ions act as crystal poisons. The concept of a crystal poison has been familiar to science for some time, but it remains a phenomenon which is not very clearly understood. The basic facts are that some compounds can inhibit the formation of crystals from supersaturated solutions by apparently settling on crystal surfaces and stopping further growth. Complex phosphate compounds appear to be particularly effective in this respect and this is in fact the basis of many of the commercial additives used as domestic water softeners. These inhibit the formation of crystals of calcium carbonate even when used in concentrations many times less than those of the calcium in the water. The effect can be visualized as involving a close fit between the phosphate complex and the calcium ions in the crystal lattice (Fig. 3–1). The phosphate groups substitute for carbonate ions in the lattice and reduce the possibility of further calcium ions being added by destroying the charge and distorting the crystal lattice. This stops crystal growth and thus favours the development of supersaturation.

On this interpretation most of the bone surfaces in the body are not continually growing even though the plasma is supersaturated for bone mineral and this is because they are coated with inhibitory pyro-phosphate ions which block the crystal lattices from further growth. The

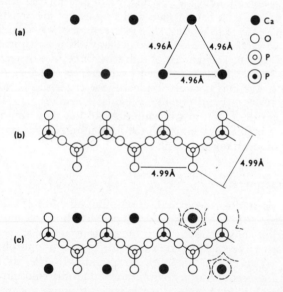

Fig. 3–1 (a) The arrangement of calcium ions in a calcite lattice. Note that each calcium ion is 4.96 Å away from its neighbour. (b) The structure of a metaphosphate ion with charged oxygen atoms being 4.99 Å apart. (c) The metaphosphate ion fitted on to the surface of a calcite crystal lattice with ionic radii shown by dotted lines. Crystal poisons may act in this way by blocking the charges and reactive sites on the surfaces of a crystal lattice so as to make further growth impossible. (10 Angstrom = 1 nm.) (Redrawn from RAISTRICK, B. (1949), *Disc. Faraday Soc.*, 5, 234–7.)

bone mineral will only continue to be formed when these 'crystal poisons' are removed or destroyed and this might account for the occurrence of amorphous deposits in newly formed bone. One of the ways these 'poisons' could be destroyed would be by hydrolysis to phosphate ions and it was suggested that this may be the function of the alkaline phosphatase which Robison found at sites of bone growth.

3.3   Later work

Alkaline phosphatase occurs at various sites of mineralization in corals, earthworms, snails, lobsters, dogfish, birds' eggshells, mammalian teeth and bones. It is tempting, therefore, to consider that in each of these cases the enzyme may be removing an inhibitor or crystal poison. Unfortunately, there is as yet little evidence to support this although inhibitors of calcification are quite common in a variety of animals' bloods and even in sea water. One of the problems which has worried people about this concept is that crystal poisons apparently only act by inhibiting the rate at which crystals and liquids come into equilibrium. Eventually, however, they would be expected to reach that stage and it is therefore not clear exactly what long-term effect they would have. Part of this problem is no doubt due to the absence of quantitative data about crystal poisons and one should, perhaps, also add that since many biological processes are extremely dynamic the final state of equilibrium may not be a critical one.

One practical use to which the concept of crystal poisons has been put is in the treatment of certain stones in the urine of patients. These people have on occasion been treated with dietary phosphate supplements which increase pyrophosphate excretion in the urine and decrease the occurrence of these painful deposits. Many of the other circumstances where crystal poisons might, however, have been expected to prove useful have been rather disappointing in their outcome. It has been suggested that this is probably because the blood and many tissues of the body possess phosphatase enzymes that can destroy complex phosphate compounds. Interest is therefore shifting at the present time to phosphonates, i.e.

$$
\begin{array}{cc}
\text{OH} & \text{OH} \\
| & | \\
\text{O}=\text{P}-\text{CH}_2-\text{P}=\text{O} \\
| & | \\
\text{OH} & \text{OH}
\end{array}
\quad\text{which are similar to pyrophosphates}\quad
\begin{array}{cc}
\text{OH} & \text{OH} \\
| & | \\
\text{O}=\text{P}-\text{O}-\text{P}=\text{O} \\
| & | \\
\text{OH} & \text{OH}
\end{array}
$$

except that there is a P–C–P bond instead of the more easily hydrolysed P–O–P linkage. This makes the phosphonates relatively stable in the body and perhaps potentially more useful in modifying the physiological process of mineralization. It remains to be seen whether this application of the concept of crystal poisons will have important medical applications.

4   Remodelling and Hormonal Control

'Improbable' means 'not likely to persist in the way described', and everything that has been said about the blood–bone relationship in the previous two chapters is improbable in physicochemical terms. The situation which has been described indicates that the blood is supersaturated with respect to bone mineral salts and that this induces crystal seeds to form on collagen fibres. The growth of crystals may be temporarily impeded by crystal poisons such as pyrophosphate ions, but it represents a non-equilibrium situation and as such would be expected to run down as it comes into equilibrium with the bone minerals.

All living systems are in a state of disequilibrium with their surroundings, however, and it is one of the basic requirements of cells that they can maintain these conditions. The blood–bone situation may not seem unreasonable, therefore, for a living system, but it means that somewhere in the body it should be possible to identify the cellular activities which are maintaining and regulating the non-equilibrium condition of the blood. The obvious place to look for such cells is in the bone itself. There are two reasons for thinking this. First, about 98 per cent of all the calcium in the mammalian body resides in the skeleton, so that this would obviously be a critical region for any overall regulation. Second, there are many reasons for thinking that the skeleton itself is in a dynamic state. If, for example, the hollow limb bone of a child simply grew by the additional deposition of minerals on its surfaces it would rapidly become a very massive and heavy structure. It is a matter of common observation that this does not happen, but that there is some compensation whereby the deposition of mineral on the outer layers of

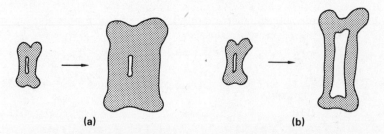

(a)   (b)

Fig. 4–1 Equal growth in all directions would produce massive heavy bones (a), whereas their proportions do not usually change very much during normal development (b). This is because the limb bones growth in length faster than in width and because the inner parts are resorbed as the bone extends.

the bone is at least partly matched by resorption from the inner layers
(Fig. 4–1). This implies that material is removed from the bone and
returned to the blood and this is the basis of bone remodelling. It is the
control of this process which is of interest to us in trying to understand
how the supersaturation of the blood is maintained. The experiment we
will discuss investigated this control system, but before considering that
we need to know a little more about the formation of bone.

4.1   Introduction

The hollow limb bones of mammals originate in the embryo as
cartilaginous structures that often appear as miniature replicas of the
adult structure. Their calcification starts with the degeneration of the
cartilage in a collar around the centre and also at the ends of the future
bone shaft. The details of the process need not concern us at the
moment, but it is important to note that the degenerating cartilage
becomes replaced by bone that is formed from special cells, the
osteoblasts. At the ends of the bones a layer of cartilage persists beneath
the bone caps or epiphyses. This cartilage continues to grow and be
replaced so that there is a persistent and rapid growth in the length of
the bone until it reaches its adult size (Fig. 4–2).

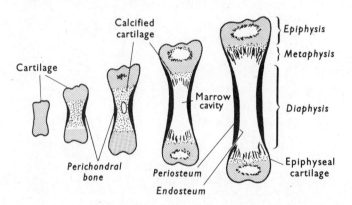

Fig. 4–2   The formation of bone in a piece of cartilage (shaded) occurs by two
different processes. Calcified cartilage (stippled) becomes eroded and eventually
replaced by layers of perichondrial bone laid down in layers from the outer
periosteal surface of the diaphysis or shaft. In mammals the ends of the bone
also retain a layer of growing cartilage which becomes converted to bone and
forms the epiphyses. Bone resorption occurs from the inner or endosteal
surfaces and the long bones characteristically grow in length much faster than
they do in width. (From SIMKISS, K. (1967), *Calcium in Reproductive Physiology*,
Chapman and Hall.)

Growth in the thickness of these bones occurs by a different mechanism. The layer of connective tissue around the original cartilage becomes modified to form a periosteum layer. This contains many osteoblasts and the bone thickens by laying down concentric sheets of bone arranged like onion skins around the shaft. Some of the osteoblast cells become surrounded by mineral and thus form the osteocyte cells which occur within the bone (Fig. 4–3).

Growth in the length of a bone occurs much faster at the epiphysial plate region than does the growth in width, so that a bone increases in size without changing its proportions. Resorption of minerals occurs mainly from the inner surface of the bone where the cells forming the endosteal layer resorb this region of the oldest part of the bone. The resorbing cells are called osteoclasts and they are very active in the endosteal region during growth. When a mammal reaches its adult size most of the growth processes cease, but bone remodelling continues in many species throughout life. The resorbing osteoclast cells now make holes through the length of the bone, forming cavities like long winding tunnels that are called Haversian canals. This localized destruction is

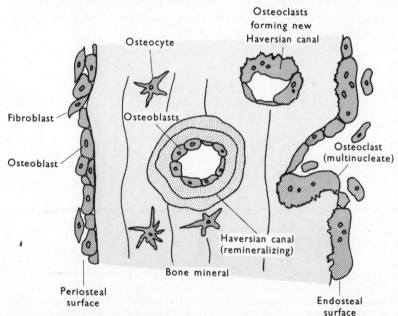

Fig. 4–3 Diagrammatic representation of a section of bone showing the main types of cells including osteoblsts (bone forming), osteocytes, and osteoclasts (resorbing). Note the outer periosteal and the inner endosteal membranes. Two Haversian canals are also shown, one being formed by osteoclasts and the other remineralized by osteoblast cells.

relatively short-lived at any one site and then the tunnel is reossified by the formation of concentric layers of bone around its walls (Fig. 4–3). Thus, throughout the life of many animals there is a continual process of tunnelling out and reossifying of the bones. This releases calcium and phosphate ions from the bone into the blood from where they are eventually excreted or redeposited in another part of the skeleton.

The amount of bone that is being remodelled can be varied. The parathyroid glands release a hormone when the calcium level of the blood falls below normal, and this hormone stimulates the osteoclast cells to resorb more bone mineral. The level of blood calcium is therefore raised, especially since the hormone also causes the kidney to allow more phosphate to be excreted from the blood and thus simultaneously decreases the possibility that bone will be reformed. As the calcium level of the blood rises the rate of secretion of parathyroid hormone slows down and bone resorption decreases. Thus the remodelling of bone provides a mechanism whereby the calcium concentration of the blood can be kept at a fairly constant and supersaturated level. This concept was generally accepted during the 1950s and it was stated in a very precise form by F. C. MCLEAN and M. URIST in 1955. They pointed out that it was a case of a typical feedback system

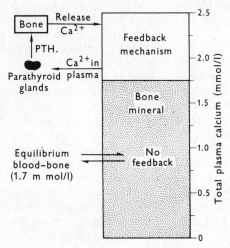

Fig. 4–4   McLean and Urist's feedback mechanism to explain the involvement of the parathyroid glands. The blood is in equilibrium with bone mineral if the plasma calcium level falls to about 1.7 mmol/l. Blood calcium is normally at a level of 2.5 mmol/l and is maintained at this level by a feedback mechanism. If the level falls below 2.5 mmol/l the parathyroid glands are stimulated to release their hormone. This causes the bone cells to resorb mineral and pass ions into the blood until the calcium level is restored to 2.5 mmol/l. (Redrawn from MCLEAN, F. C. and URIST, M. R. (1968), *Bone,* 3rd edn., Univ. Chicago Press.)

of control. Any variation in the level of blood calcium affected the parathyroid glands whose secretion induced changes in the body until this 'feedback' brought the change in blood calcium level back to normal (Fig. 4–4). This clear statement of the current theories caused a number of people to consider whether the system of calcium control really was so simple. If it was, how could the level of plasma calcium be regulated if there was too much calcium in the blood instead of too little? According to MCLEAN the excess of calcium simply caused a cessation in the secretion of parathyroid hormone so that bone resorption decreased, presumably until the excess calcium was excreted or deposited in bone. Some opinions were voiced that this was too crude a control system, and that it would lead to oscillations in the blood calcium levels as the parathyroid glands were continually turned on and off. It was at this stage that H. D. COPP decided to try to investigate the control of the parathyroid gland over the levels of calcium in the blood.

4.2 The experiment

In 1962 COPP, CAMERON, CHENEY, DAVIDSON and HENZE published the results of their experiments in which they modified the normal calcium levels in the blood of dogs. A simplified form of the experimental system they used is shown in Fig. 4–5. Dogs were fasted overnight and then anaesthetized with a barbiturate injection. A second injection of an anticoagulant, heparin, was given to stop blood clotting. A small plastic tube or cannula was then inserted into the carotid artery in the neck region and blood was circulated from there into the superior thyroid artery by means of a peristaltic perfusion pump. The speed of the pump was controlled so as to keep the blood pressure at about 120–150 mm Hg. This was checked by means of manometers in the normal and perfused circulation to ensure that the animal maintained a normal blood pressure. The flow of blood through the parathyroid and thyroid glands was controlled by the perfusion pump while the glands were removed from the body and placed in a moist chamber kept at 38°C. The blood leaving the glands was collected into another cannula tube and passed into the body via the jugular vein. Thus the thyroid and parathyroid glands were isolated from the body, but still remained within the blood circulation of the dog. A small tap was fixed into the plastic tubing carrying blood to the isolated glands and during an experiment calcium chloride solution was pumped into this so as to raise the level of calcium in the blood entering the glands by 0.5 mmol/l. In an alternative experiment the compound ethylene diamine tetraacetic acid (EDTA) was made up in solution and added at an equivalent rate. This compound binds calcium ions very strongly into a non-toxic compound so that it was then possible to lower the level of ionic plasma calcium by 0.5 mmol/l. The actual amount of calcium infused was 5 to

12.5 μmol/kg body wt/h, but the experiment was so arranged that a calcium infusion for 1 to 2 hours was always followed by an EDTA infusion for a similar period. Thus the total amount of ionic calcium added to the dog at one time was identical to the quantity removed later.

In this experiment, COPP and his colleagues were trying to investigate whether hormones released from the thyroid and parathyroid glands influenced the level of calcium in the blood. In order to stimulate the glands they had to vary the concentration of calcium in the blood entering the glands, but they did not want this treatment to confuse their

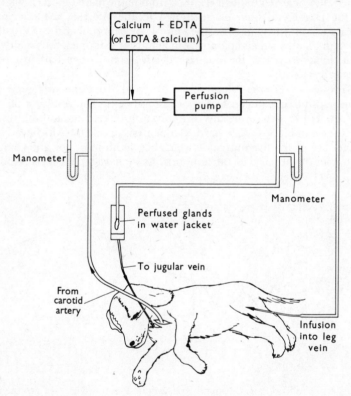

Fig. 4-5 The experimental system used in the discovery of the hormone calcitonin. The thyroid and parathyroid glands were isolated from the body but perfused with blood from the carotid artery of the dog. Calcium was added or removed from the blood going to the glands, but a correcting treatment enabled calcium to be removed or added to blood passing into the leg vein so that no overall changes were caused. Blood which had perfused the endocrine glands and which contained their hormones re-entered the dog via the jugular vein. (Modified from COPP, D. H. and DAVIDSON, A. G. F. (1961), *Proc. Soc. exp. Biol. Med.*, **107**, 342–4.)

results. They were careful to ensure, therefore, that any extra calcium added to the blood to stimulate the glands was removed when it entered the general circulation by adding an equivalent amount of EDTA into a vein in the leg. Similarly, when EDTA was added to the blood perfused through the glands they added an equivalent amount of calcium into the leg vein. Thus although they varied the calcium level of the blood passing through the glands great care was taken to ensure that they compensated for this so that the level of calcium ions in the rest of the circulation was not affected by the experimental treatment. Any changes which they detected in the level of calcium in the main blood circulation of the dog could then be attributed to the effect of the hormones released from the glands. At the end of the experiment the circulation through the thyroid and parathyroid glands was stopped, thus removing their influence from the dog as effectively as if they had just been surgically cut out.

Samples of arterial blood were collected from the dog every 15 minutes and centrifuged to remove blood cells. The resulting plasma was titrated to determine the concentration of calcium and the results are shown in Fig. 4–6. The particular analysis of calcium which was used makes use of the dye murexide which acts as an indicator and changes colour in the absence of calcium ions. As we have seen, EDTA removes

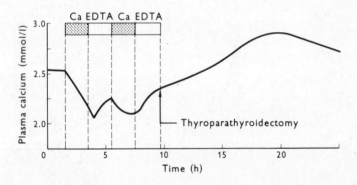

Fig. 4–6   Results obtained using the technique shown in Fig. 4–5. For the first 10 h the animal behaved as if the calcium level of the blood was controlled by the parathyroid glands. Addition of calcium caused a decrease in parathyroid hormone secretion and a fall in plasma calcium levels. Removing calcium stimulated the parathyroid gland and raised plasma calcium levels. After 10 h the endocrine glands were removed from the circulation. It was expected that this would cause a fall in blood calcium due to the loss of parathyroid hormone. The rise in blood calcium levels could only be explained by invoking the loss of a new hormone—calcitonin. (Modified from COPP, D. H., CAMERON, E. C., CHENEY, B. A., DAVIDSON, A. G. F. and HENZE, E. G. (1962), *Endocrinology,* **70**, 638–49.)

calcium ions by binding them into a complex compound, and it was therefore used to titrate the plasma until the indicator changed colour. The quantity of EDTA added was then equivalent to the amount of calcium ions originally present. Note that this is rather a clever experimental trick because EDTA has already been used to change the level of calcium ions in the perfused blood. By using the same compound to analyse the blood for free calcium these workers automatically ensured that the calcium ions already removed by the EDTA given to the dog would not be detected in the analysis.

4.3   Discussion

Experiments on live animals should only be undertaken with great care, humanity and thought. In Great Britain there are strict laws controlling such operations, and the scientific world imposes its own standards to ensure that cruelty or careless acts are not tolerated. Wherever possible, experiments are performed under anaesthesia and the animals are normally killed while in this state so that no pain is experienced. The work of COPP and his co-workers in Canada was of this standard. In addition to the ethical problems, however, a great number of physiological safeguards have also to be checked to ensure that the results obtained are relevant to normal healthy animals. Thus, the highest standards of surgery are necessary to ensure that the animals do not bleed excessively or experience surgical shock. This is one of the reasons why the blood pressure of the dog was measured continuously and why the blood pressure in the perfusion system was kept at the same level by means of a pump. Many organs would cease to function normally if the blood pressure fell, and it was important in this experiment that the isolated glands were kept as responsive as possible. For the same reason the glands were perfused in a thermostated water bath at the same temperature as the dog's body.

The four parathyroid glands of a dog are extremely small and only weigh about 1 g altogether. They lie very close to and partly embedded in the much larger thyroid glands of the neck and in order to simplify the surgery it was decided not to try and separate them but to perfuse the two sets of glands together through a common artery. This decision was to have enormous implications as we will see later.

Animals possess very efficient homeostatic systems. If something is damaged or changed the body will often compensate for it by effecting its own adjustments, and this makes physiological experiments very demanding in their design and interpretation. This particular experiment involved circulating blood through isolated glands, but as soon as a blood vessel is cut compensatory changes occur which tend to seal off that region by clotting the blood. If these changes were allowed to occur it would be very difficult to pass blood out of the blood vessels and through the glands of the dog, and for this reason heparin was injected into the dog. Heparin is a polysaccharide material which stops the blood from clotting and, therefore, makes it easier to perfuse tissues. It is similarly often very difficult to influence one part of an animal without upsetting the whole organism. This is the reason the experimental plan was so complex, for all that COPP wished to do was to see whether stimulating the glands, by giving them a deficiency of calcium, made the body compensate by releasing calcium from the dog's bones. In order to do this, however, they had to ensure that the experimental stimulus (i.e. low levels of plasma calcium) did not contaminate the response that was being measured (i.e. level of plasma calcium). This was cleverly done by means of an exactly equivalent injection of calcium into the leg vein which balanced out the effect of the EDTA given to the perfused glands. This may seem a complicated procedure, but it is typical of the types of technique that are necessary to isolate the usually very well integrated 'cause and effect' reactions found in biology.

One final comment should perhaps be added about the technique. It will be noticed that the dogs were not fed before the experiment. This is partly because it makes surgery safer, by reducing the possibility of vomiting, but also because if a dog had recently eaten, there may be an absorption of calcium from the intestine during the operation. This could lead to a steadily rising level of blood calcium which would make the interpretation of the work difficult. Biological experiments often show a lot of variation between individual specimens even when the experimental conditions are carefully controlled. For this reason statistics are normally used to investigate mathematically the degree of variation due to the treatments, as opposed to that due to individual differences. This mathematical analysis was performed by COPP but in addition they used another technique in which they reversed the treatment during an experiment to check that the animal's reactions also reversed. By doing this they were able to use the same animal as virtually its own control, as can be seen from the results of the typical experiment shown in Fig. 4–6.

4.4 The interpretation

The experiment was originally devised to test McLean's hypothesis that the calcium level of the blood was regulated by a feedback system involving the parathyroid glands. A high calcium concentration in the blood should reduce the rate of hormone secretion, reduce the rate of bone resorption and thus lower the plasma calcium level. Low calcium concentrations would stimulate the parathyroids and thus lead to an elevated level of blood calcium. It can be clearly seen from Fig. 4–6 that this is exactly what did happen in the first half of the experiment and, in fact, these workers originally reported in 1961 that their experiments provided good support for McLean's hypothesis. Fortunately, however, they did not stop their experiments there. It is difficult to explain why they performed the next procedure, except that previously they had tried varying the conditions at the end of an experiment and had observed some strange results. A decade later COPP still had difficulty explaining just why he did the experiment.

'In 1957 we were carrying out a prolonged infusion of EDTA in a dog, and, *for some reason*, performed a thyroparathyroidectomy at the end of the infusion. To our consternation the plasma calcium immediately rose above normal—a most unorthodox response to the removal of the parathyroids!' (COPP, COCKCROFT, KUEH and MELVILLE, 1968.)

In fact it is likely that the removal of the thyroid and parathyroid glands was not part of the original experiment, but was included at the end as a check on the technique. The results so surprised the experimenters that they did not publish them for six years. In the meantime, however, they did not discard the strange data, but repeated the observations in other circumstances. The second half of the experiment we have described was just such an occasion. Note the situation in that up until 10 h of experimentation everything is in keeping with the concept that the release of parathyroid hormone produces a rise in plasma calcium levels. In the second half of the experiment, however, the thyroid and parathyroid glands were removed, but instead of this leading to a fall in blood calcium levels they rose sharply and remained high for many hours. This was an extremely strange and unexpected response that could not be explained by the existing theories of the control of blood calcium and parathyroid function. The only way to explain the data was to suggest that there must be another hormone secreted from the same perfused glands but with the exact opposite effects of parathyroid hormone. This new hormone was called calcitonin and COPP suggested that its main effect was to cause a lowering of plasma calcium levels. It appeared, therefore, to be an antagonist to parathyroid hormone which if removed allowed the blood calcium level to rise.

4.5 Later work

In the decade since the calcitonin hypothesis was first proposed a great deal of work has been devoted to isolating and studying the properties of this hormone. The hormone is produced by a group of cells associated with the terminal gill of the embryo. In mammals these cells migrate during development and eventually become incorporated as the so-called c cells of the thyroid. It was this fortuitous association which led, as we have seen, to their discovery in a preparation originally devised to study parathyroid functions. In non-mammalian vertebrates the calcitonin secreting cells often remain distinct as a small ultimobranchial gland (Fig. 4–7).

Calcitonin is released in increasing quantities as the plasma calcium level rises. Parathyroid hormone is released as the hormone concentration falls (Fig. 4–8). The two hormones are thus released in exactly opposite situations. The minimal secretion rates of both hormones

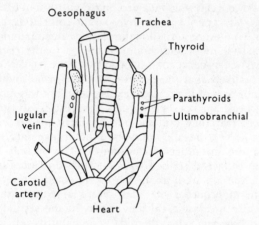

Fig. 4–7   The thyroid, parathyroid and ultimobranchial glands as seen in a dissection of the neck region of the fowl.

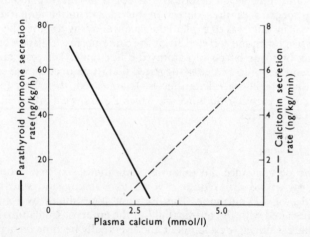

Fig. 4–8   The rates of secretion of parathyroid and calcitonin hormones at different plasma calcium levels. (Data for various mammals from COPP, D. H. (1969), *J. Endocrin.*, **43**, 137–61.)

occur at the normal blood calcium levels of about 2.5 mmol/l. Since only part of the total calcium in the blood is dissociated, this corresponds with a level of ionic calcium of about 1.67 mmol/l which is the level used by NEUMAN in his demonstration that the blood was supersaturated (Chapter 2). It appears, therefore, that this supersaturated state corresponds to the set point in the interplay of calcitonin and parathyroid hormone and this interpretation is supported by the observation that removal of the parathyroid glands causes the plasma calcium level to fall to about 70 per cent of its normal value, i.e. to the level at which it is in equilibrium with bone mineral (Fig. 4–4). In the mammal both hormones appear to influence bone resorption; calcitonin by inhibiting it, and parathyroid hormone by stimulating it. In other vertebrates the control system may be somewhat different since it is difficult to demonstrate that calcitonin produces much of a response when injected into birds or fish. Both these groups of animals produce their own secretions of calcitonin but it may be that it influences other target organs in the body.

One of the surprising aspects of the hormonal control of calcium metabolism is the fact that the rate of secretion of both parathyroid hormone and calcitonin is directly proportional to the variation of plasma calcium levels (Fig. 4–8). One would perhaps have expected a control system which responded more rapidly the greater the deviation from normal plasma levels. Such a type of system is called a derivative control system and it has the advantages that it tends to respond faster to large deviations but slower as the system returns to normal. In this way it avoids overshooting the return to normal values. The problem of overcompensating for a disturbance in the physiology of an animal may also be avoided by having antagonists which damp down the responses of the system. This appears to be what calcitonin does to the parathyroid response in mammals.

Finally, it is worth noting that the vertebrate skeletal system is unusual in having cells dispersed through it which enable the continual remodelling of the bones. The skeletons of other animals are often calcified and some, like those of the decapod crustacea are often decalcified before they are discarded during a moult. The calcium is then stored and later used to recalcify the new skeleton. Some molluscs decalcify the shell during periods of anoxia or acidosis and presumably recalcify the resorbed regions later. In none of these situations is there any known mechanism for regulating the remodelling of the skeleton in the way that vertebrates do. In fact, although there is evidence for the regulation of calcium metabolism in invertebrates almost nothing is known about its hormonal control. It is therefore difficult to draw comparisons with the vertebrate system, although it is worth noting the enormous possibilities for such studies among the invertebrates.

5 Kinetic Studies

The concept that the skeleton is a stable, inert structure became untenable when radioisotopes were introduced into biological research. The ionizing radiations which these isotopes emit made it possible for scientists to detect where they accumulated in the skeleton, and it soon became apparent that bone was a very varied and dynamic material. Thus new mineral might be deposited in one region of a bone due to growth, remodelling or repair while an adjacent site might be in the process of being resorbed in response to a calcium deficient diet or the strain of lactation. The problem was to find a way of measuring these activities when they varied so much from region to region and were spread throughout such a massive organ.

The classical method of measuring calcium metabolism is the balance experiment. In this technique the food which a person eats is weighed and analysed so that its calcium content can be estimated. The urine and faeces are collected and similarly weighed and analysed so as to assess the calcium loss. Subtracting these two values makes it possible to determine whether the body is gaining or losing calcium. Unfortunately, this net value may obscure all sorts of variations. If a man resorbs 2 g of calcium from his skeleton every day but simultaneously remineralizes an equivalent amount of his bones he will appear to be in normal calcium balance, even though his rate of bone formation and destruction is four times normal. As such he is probably suffering from a disturbance of his parathyroid glands, but in order to diagnose this accurately it would be valuable to know his bone formation and resorption rates.

One of the techniques which has been developed for investigating problems of this sort is called 'compartmental analysis'. It is a method that is particularly well suited to the use of radioisotopes, for it attempts to study the behaviour in the body of some relevant substance, such as ^{45}Ca, and explain this in terms of abstract functions. By manipulating the data in experiments of this sort it is often possible to isolate particular expressions which refer to the problem in hand. The method will, however, be best understood if we look at the way it developed in the study of bones and then take a specific example.

In 1948 NORRIS and KISIELESKI reported some experiments in which they injected radioactive calcium into rats. Samples of blood were taken at various times after the injection and analysed for radioactive calcium (^{45}Ca) and total calcium ($^{40}Ca + ^{45}Ca$). The ratio of these two measurements (i.e. $^{45}Ca/^{40}Ca + ^{45}Ca$) is called the specific activity, since it indicates how much of the total calcium is associated with the radioactive label. For this reason NORRIS and KISIELESKI also measured the specific activity of the skeleton, expecting that only a thin film of radioisotope would occur over the bones, which would therefore have a very low specific activity. As the experiment progressed the specific activity of the blood decreased as the ^{45}Ca was excreted from the body and replaced by normal dietary calcium. It was confidently expected that the specific activity of the skeleton would follow a similar trend as the radioisotope 'washed off' the outermost crystals of the skeleton to which it had become temporarily attached. In fact these expectations were not upheld, for although the specific activity of the blood fell rapidly, that of the skeleton remained high and on the tenth day of the experiment was actually higher than that of the blood. Clearly the isotope was being retained in the skeleton as more than just a film over the surface of the bones and NORRIS and KISIELESKI concluded 'This seems to indicate that certain physical and/or metabolic factors are involved which prevent the overall picture from being that of a simple equilibria and exchange as it is ordinarily considered.'

One must assume that in 1948 it was difficult for people to envisage that the skeleton was anything but an inert structure. By 1955, however, a number of scientists had recognized that what NORRIS and KISIELESKI'S experiment demonstrated was that new bone was continually being formed and thus radioisotopes were being trapped and deposited away from contact with the blood. In fact the Swedish scientists BAUER, CARLSSON and LINDQUIST saw even greater implications in the work. They realized that if the quantity of radioisotope which was trapped by bone growth could somehow be separated from that associated with the outermost surfaces of the skeleton then they would have a measure of the rate of deposition of new bone. Accordingly, they set out to try and separate the various influences involved in incorporating radioisotopes into bone.

5.1   The experiments

The experiments were performed on three-month-old rats which were kept in individual cages and fed a normal but uniform diet. The animals were divided into ten groups each of four rats, with care being taken to make the effects of litter, sex and weight equal throughout the groups. Each rat was then injected at 9 a.m. with 1 ml of saline containing 15 μCi of ^{45}Ca. The injection was made into the body cavity of the rats and the groups of animals were then killed at carefully spaced times of from 15 min to 48 h.

The rats were anaesthetized with ether before they were killed and a large blood sample was taken. This was allowed to clot and the remaining serum was titrated to determine its calcium content. The titrated sample was then stored for later radioactive measurements. The ends and shaft of the left tibio-fibula bones were removed and cleaned of as much tissue and blood as possible. They were placed in a muffle furnace and heated at 500°C for 24 h to remove all organic material and convert them to ash. The ash was dissolved in.acid and titrated to determine its calcium content. The titrated samples were again stored for radioactive measurements later.

The amount of radioactivity in a sample is a property which continually changes as it 'decays'. The rate of decay is not affected by such variables as temperature or pressure so that it is very predictable but it is obviously of great importance to 'count' the radioactivity at a known time so that compensation can be made for the amount of decay.

In the case of ^{45}Ca the half life is 165 days which means that 165 days after the experiment starts the amount of radioactivity will have declined to half its original value irrespective of experimental treatments. The radioactivity of the calcium samples was therefore measured at known times by means of a Geiger–Muller tube. These tubes separate large electrical potential differences and respond to the ionizing radiations of radioisotopes by allowing a transient conduction of electricity. The number of such electric discharges are recorded as a measure of the radioactivity of the samples.

The change in blood specific activity during this experiment is shown in Fig. 5–1 and the changes in bone radioactivity are illustrated in Fig. 5–2.

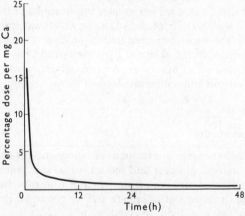

Fig. 5–1 The change of specific activity in the blood of rats after a single injection of ^{45}Ca. (Data from BAUER, G. H., CARLSSON, A. and LINDQUIST, B. (1955), *Acta Physiol. Scand.*, **35**, 56–66.)

5.2 Discussion and results

The results obtained by BAUER, CARLSSON and LINDQUIST were basically rather simple. It will be apparent that they took the usual experimental

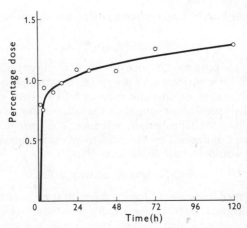

Fig. 5–2 The accumulation of ^{45}Ca in the shafts of the tibias of rats after a single injection of isotope. (Data from BAUER, G. H., CARLSSON, A. and LINDQUIST, B. (1961), *Mineral Metabolism,* Vol. 1B, Academic Press.)

precautions of controlling the diet, types of animal and sites of injection. In addition, there are some health problems in working with radioactive substances so that great care has to be exercised to ensure that no radioactivity is absorbed by the experimenter or allowed to contaminate working regions. Radioactive counting must be checked to ensure that compensation is made for any decay with time and there are also complex instrumental problems. Sometimes the non-radioactive material in a sample will absorb much of the radiation produced so that the counting equipment only detects a fraction of the radioactivity present. Similarly, the equipment may only be capable of responding quickly enough to detect a fraction of the radiation it receives over any period of time. Both these problems can be overcome by using suitable controls and by accepting that the readings obtained are simply proportional to the total radiation present in the samples (detected as counts/min) rather than measuring it all (which would be disintegrations/min).

The exciting aspect of these experiments is, however, the series of bold postulates which BAUER, CARLSSON and LINDQUIST made for their interpretation. They argued that there were only two ways that radioactive calcium ions could enter bone. In the first process the surfaces of non-growing regions of the bone could exchange ions with the blood so that some ^{45}Ca would become associated with the mineral faces. In growing regions of the bone the second mechanism would also apply by the deposition of new mineral from the various calcium ions in the blood. These processes of calcium exchange (^{45}Ca$_E$) and calcium accretion (^{45}Ca$_A$) should therefore account for all the radioactivity observed in the bone ($^{45}Ca_{obs}$) provided that there was no bone resorption, i.e.

$$^{45}Ca_{obs} = {}^{45}Ca_E + {}^{45}Ca_A \qquad (1)$$

In order to pursue this analysis they then postulated that the exchangeable bone surfaces were always in contact with the blood. Thus at any single instant of time the ratio of ^{45}Ca to total calcium in the exchangeable bone fraction would be the same as that in the blood, i.e. they would have the same specific activities. The specific activity of the blood at time t multiplied by the quantity of exchangeable bone in the skeleton (E) would thus define the value $^{45}Ca_E$, i.e.

$$^{45}Ca_E = (\text{specific activity})_t \times E.$$

Newly-formed bone would have a different specific activity since that which was formed early in the experiment would contain a lot of radioisotope, whereas that formed later would contain less ^{45}Ca. In other words, the specific activity of newly-formed bone would tend to be more like the average specific activity of the blood during the period of the experiment. This value multiplied by the duration of the experiment and the rate of new bone formation (A) would thus define the value $^{45}Ca_A$, i.e.

$$^{45}Ca_A = (\text{mean specific activity}) \times t \times A.$$

The change in serum specific activity is usually obtained by taking the area beneath the specific activity curve between the start and end of the experiment or by integrating the curve over the same time period, i.e.

$$\int_0^t \text{Sp. Act. } (t) \ dt.$$

The important point to note is that exchangeable bone (E) will have a specific activity equal to that of the blood *at the time when the bone sample is taken* whereas the newly formed bone (A) will have a specific activity represented by the *mean specific activity throughout the experiment*. This enables E and A to be separated since equation (1) now becomes

$$^{45}Ca_{obs} = [(\text{Sp. Act})_t \times E] + [\int_0^t \text{Sp. Act. } (t) \ dt \times A]$$

This equation contains two variables that can be measured, i.e. the total radioactivity in the bone ($^{45}Ca_{obs}$) and the specific activity of the serum at various times. It has also two constants E and A which can, therefore, be determined from the results obtained at different time intervals by the use of simultaneous equations. 'E', of course, represents the mass of bone available for exchange with the blood and 'A' measures the rate of formation of new bone.

When the results obtained from the shafts of the rat bones were analysed in this way the graphs shown in Fig. 5–3 were obtained. It will be apparent that when the curves for E and A are added together they

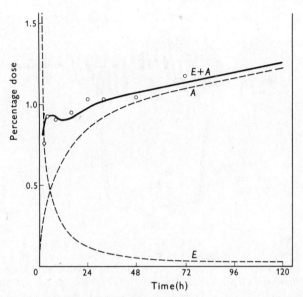

Fig. 5–3 The exchangeable (E) and newly formed (A) fractions of bone in the diaphysis of rat tibias calculated from radio-isotope studies. The circles (○) show the actual observed distribution of ^{45}Ca determined experimentally and there is a close fit with the calculated curve $E + A$. (After BAUER, G. H., CARLSSON, A. and LINDQUIST, B. (1961), *Mineral Metabolism,* Vol. 1B, Academic Press.)

provide a very good fit for the experimental data, indicating that they account for all the radioisotope actually observed in the bones.

When the experiments were repeated on the·epiphyseal ends of the bones, however, there was a large discrepancy between the experimental data and the curves E and A. It will be recalled, that the epiphyses grow much faster than the shaft of the bone. It appeared likely, therefore, that in the 10 days of the experiment the epiphysis would have grown so much on the outer surface and been resorbed so fast from the inner surface that the original radioactive label would have passed through the bone and been released from the endosteal surface (Fig. 5–4). Thus the ^{45}Ca$_{obs}$ will be less than ^{45}Ca$_E$ + ^{45}Ca$_A$ by the amount of this resorption (^{45}Ca$_R$), i.e.

$$^{45}\text{Ca}_{obs} = {}^{45}\text{Ca}_A + {}^{45}\text{Ca}_E - {}^{45}\text{Ca}_R$$

Thus, the difference between the observed data and 'accretion plus exchange' can be plotted as resorption (Fig. 5–5). By this means it is possible to obtain estimates of the rates of bone accretion and resorption and of the size of the exchangeable fraction of bone. These results are shown in Table 5–1 for the epiphyses, shafts and whole tibias of rats.

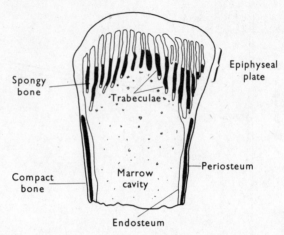

Fig. 5–4 The distribution of ^{45}Ca in a section of a long bone of a rat 1 week after a single injection of the isotope. Radioactivity is shown by a thick line. Note how the radioactivity has become covered over by the deposition of new bone. The growth of the epiphyseal plate is so fast that the isotope has almost reached the endosteal surface and will therefore be resorbed in the next 1–2 days.

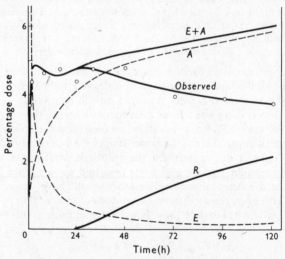

Fig. 5–5 A similar experiment to the one shown in Fig. 5–3 except that measurements are made on the epiphyses instead of the shaft of the bone. The experimentally-observed data (o) no longer fits the curve $E + A$ since some of the isotope has been resorbed in this rapidly growing region of the bone (cf. Fig. 5–4). The difference between the observed data and the curve $E + A$ is, therefore, represented by R (bone resorption). (After BAUER, G. H., CARLSSON, A. and LINDQUIST, B. (1961), *Mineral Metabolism*, Vol. 1B, Academic Press.)

Table 5–1   Calcium metabolism in the tibias of rats assessed by kinetic studies with ^{45}Ca. (Data from BAUER, G. H., CARLSSON, A., and LINDQUIST, B. (1955), *K. fysiogr Sallsk. Lund. Forh.*, **25**, 3–18.)

	Whole tibia	Ends (epiphyses)	Shafts
Calcium content (mg)	66	36	30
Accretion (mg Ca/h)	0.17	0.14	0.03
Resorption (mg Ca/h)	0.13	0.12	0.01
Exchangeable fraction (mg Ca)	2.0	1.7	0.3

5·3   The interpretation

Traditionally, biologists are very concerned with structures. Dissection, anatomy and histology are the bases of most biologists' training and the functions performed by animals are usually thought of as being related to particular structures. Thus, the blood is circulated by the heart and urine is produced by the kidneys. There are good reasons for maintaining these approaches to our understanding of animals, but it should be recognized that the method has its limitations and that there are alternatives. One of these is the technique of making mathematical models which simulate biological phenomena. This is done without any reference to the organs involved or to the anatomy of the animal concerned. The isotope disappearance curve shown in Fig. 5–1 can be reproduced mathematically as a sum of exponentials, i.e.

$$\text{plasma specific activity} = Ae^{-\alpha t} + Be^{-\beta t}$$

It is then possible to solve these equations by knowing the values of the constant e and time t and thus obtain numerical values for A, B, α and β which describe this particular biological phenomenon. These values cannot be related to normal biological concepts, but that is no barrier to their use. If, for example, it can be shown that a certain disease or drug has a large effect upon one of these values, then the method provides a most valuable tool for investigating the effect further. The analysis which BAUER, CARLSSON and LINDQUIST used was rather unusual in that they tried to define their mathematical values in terms of the biological concepts of bone formation, resorption and exchange. It has been criticized for this reason and it has been suggested, for example, that their values of E and A are not independent of each other. It remains, however, as a most useful and ingenious analysis which initiated a whole new system of experimentation in calcified tissues. In recent years the technique has been used on human patients with hormonal disturbances, on domestic fowl during the process of eggshell formation and on rachitic rats with and without vitamin D therapy. Some typical changes in the rates of bone formation and resorption during these treatments are shown in Table 5–2.

Compartmental analysis may be useful in its own right, but there are other reasons for using these mathematical approaches to define functions or 'compartments' in animals. One of these is that not all biological phenomena can be defined anatomically. Thus the idea of 'exchangeable' bone means 'that region of the bone which can exchange ions with the blood'. There is undoubtedly an anatomical association with such regions, but they are defined as regions where exchange occurs and as such they should be measured in this way. Unfortunately, there may be no way of knowing which parts of the skeleton exist in this form and certainly no way of sampling or measuring them in the intact animal without using a technique such as compartmental analysis.

Table 5–2 The variations in bone metabolism detected in humans suffering from parathyroid hormone disturbances and in rachitic rats before and after receiving vitamin D treatment. (Data from BAUER, G. H., CARLSSON, A. and LINDQUIST, B. (1961) in *Mineral Metabolism*, Vol. 1B, ed. COMAR, C. L. and BRONNER, F. Academic Press, pp. 341–444.)

	Accretion (g Ca/d)	Resorption (g Ca/d)	Exchangeable Ca (g Ca)
Hyperparathyroid human before operation	2.2	2.2	7.8
Hyperparathyroid human after operation	1.0	0	6.6
Rachitic rat before vitamin treatment	0.001	0.001	0.014
Rachitic rat after treatment	0.003	0.002	0.025

5.4   Later work

Out of experiments such as the one just described has come the recognition that the skeleton is continually being formed and resorbed and this has had many important consequences. The replacement of the skeleton is virtually 100 per cent in the first year of human life so that the young are very likely to accumulate bone-seeking contaminants from the environment, and in the late 1950s concern was expressed that this was exactly what was happening. The proliferation of nuclear bomb explosions led to the release of the radioactive element ^{90}Sr into the atmosphere and this inevitably became ingested and incorporated into

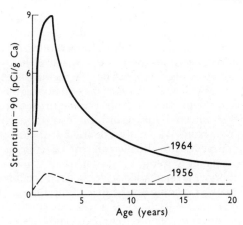

Fig. 5–6   The concentration of ^{90}Sr in the bones of humans living in Great Britain in 1956 and 1964. (Data from FLETCHER, W., LOUTIT, J. F. and PAPWORTH, D. G. (1966), *Br. Med. J.*, **2**, 1225–30.)

the skeleton. By 1964 it had reached levels which were causing alarm throughout the world (Fig. 5–6), but fortunately the signing of the Partial Test Ban Treaty in August 1963 has led to a decline in levels since that time.

In the adult there is usually about 3–5 per cent of the skeleton undergoing active accretion and resorption at any one time, and as we have seen a number of hormones can influence this. In addition, mechanical stress and pressure appears to influence the kinetics of calcium metabolism. Thus, confinement to bed for long periods, especially with immobilizing diseases such as poliomyelitis, leads to a dramatic loss in bone mass. The same phenomenon occurs in astronauts where the problem of weightlessness may lead to over 10 per cent of the skeleton being demineralized within a few weeks unless special exercises are arranged to stress the skeletal system. It has been claimed that one of the reasons for this is that bone is a piezoelectric material. Piezoelectric phenomena are associated with certain crystals which lack a centre of symmetry. When these crystals are mechanically deformed positive and negative charges are separated and appear on opposite faces of the crystals. A voltage can therefore be detected across the crystal and this phenomenon is used in the 'pick up' heads of some electric gramophones so as to convert the mechanical movements of the needle into the electrical signals that are amplified and played through the loudspeaker. A number of scientists in Japan and the U.S.A. showed in the 1950s that electrical potentials were produced when bone was bent, and perhaps the best demonstration of this was by BASSETT and BECKER in

1962 (Fig. 5–7). They clearly showed that the concave side of a bent piece of bone became negatively charged and then went on to implant small electric batteries into the bones of dogs for several weeks. They claimed that at the end of this time there was a massive deposition of bone around the cathode or negative electrode. According to their theory it is necessary continually to stress the skeletal system because the bone cells are stimulated by the piezoelectric effects that are then produced. In the absence of these effects bone resorption exceeds accretion and the skeleton becomes resorbed as in invalids and astronauts.

One of the attractions of the piezoelectric effect is that it goes some way towards explaining Wolff's Law of 1892. This states that the components of bones arrange themselves in the direction of stresses and modify their mass in relation to the deforming forces. In other words bone material arranges itself so as to be thicker in weight-bearing regions and thinner in regions that carry no stress. The bones of crippled people or of athletes differ from those of other individuals because of these responses. The advocates of the piezoelectric theory would claim that this is because the bone cells respond to the electric effects produced during exercise. Underlying the whole phenomenon, however, is the rapid turnover of the bone minerals. The fact that one can now think in these terms is due to the demonstration of accretion and resorption and the general dynamic state of the skeletal system. This most important development has arisen from the use of radioisotopes in biology and in the mathematical skill of interpreting the movements of these substances about the body.

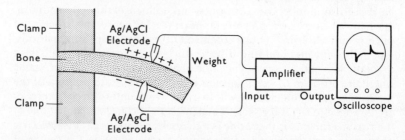

Fig. 5–7 Piezoelectric phenomena can be recorded from a piece of bone by clamping it at one end and applying weights to the free end. Silver/silver chloride electrodes are attached to upper and lower surfaces and the potential differences are amplified and displayed on an oscilloscope. The stretched surface of the bone becomes positively charged relative to the compressed side. The results shown on the oscilloscope are those that would be obtained by adding and removing a weight.

6 Cellular Aspects and Conclusions

In Fig. 6–1 an attempt has been made to summarize the main conclusions which have been drawn from the experiments described in this book. It shows the body fluids as supersaturated for bone mineral so that bone accretion is occurring on the epitactic surface of collagen fibres. Crystal poisons prevent the uncontrolled formation of mineral which is therefore restricted to the region of the osteoblast cells which destroy these inhibitors by secreting the enzyme alkaline phosphatase. Bone resorption occurs in the presence of the osteoclast cells and this process returns calcium and phosphate ions to the blood, thereby keeping it supersaturated. The balance between bone accretion and bone resorption is maintained by the actions of these cells, controlled by a feedback system involving calcitonin and parathyroid hormone. It is possible to measure this balance in the turnover rate of bone mineral by using radioisotopes and suitable kinetic studies. The value of Fig. 6–1 is that it is a shorthand way of reminding one of the data obtained from the four previous experiments. The danger is that it takes on a reality of its own which is quite unjustified, as we will shortly see.

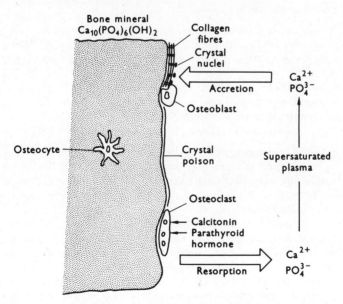

Fig. 6–1 Factors influencing the formation and resorption of bone.

The final scientific publication which we will discuss in this book differs from the ones so far considered in that it is more concerned with concepts than with individual results. Again, in order to appreciate it, one needs to look at the growth of an idea, and in particular, at a man standing up in public and stating honestly that his work does not seem to agree with current ideas.

6.1   Introduction

In 1955 JOHN E. HOWARD gave a paper at a scientific meeting organized by CIBA on the subject of *Bone Structure and Metabolism*. In this talk he gave his views as a clinician on the problems of interpreting the results he obtained from his patients in terms of the generally accepted theories of parathyroid function. In particular, the composition of their blood seemed to bear no relationship to the solubility of bone minerals. He concluded 'it is difficult to escape the concept that the relationship is guarded and supervised by a living mechanism and that it is upon such a system that parathyroid hormone . . . acts. One visualizes, therefore, a living barrier between the interstitial fluid (of bone) and the tissues of the body.'

It must be admitted that in his talk HOWARD gave little direct evidence for a cellular membrane around bone and the idea was unorthodox in the extreme. It was not surprising, therefore, that at the end of his talk the following questions were asked:

Q. 'Your postulate about a membrane, or rather your postulate about a physiochemical mechanism is most welcome to me. . . . When you then go on to a histological basis and try to show a membrane I am not with you. . . .'

Q. 'I would like to thank Dr. Howard for what I think is a tremendously helpful concept. Could we not imagine, however, that this is a theoretical membrane?'

Q. 'You still maintain that there is a membrane around bone?'

The bone membrane concept lay fallow for the next twelve years, during which time the generally accepted idea was that the blood and bone minerals were in intimate contact. Slowly, however, a variety of problems arose, and the first of these came rather unexpectedly from studies of intracellular calcium.

The enormous interest in muscle physiology in the 1960s led to a number of investigations on the role of intracellular calcium in controlling the contractile process. The best estimates indicated that normally intracellular calcium must be at a concentration of about 10^{-5} mmol/l in order for the muscle to relax. Analyses of the movement of calcium in the axoplasm of nerves gave similar results and it became generally accepted that most cells contained very little calcium in their cytoplasm. Apparently, there is a difference of several thousand-fold between the concentration of calcium in the body fluids (2.5 mmol/l) and that of the cell interior (10^{-3} mmol/l).

A few years later A. BORLE undertook a kinetic study of the rate of calcium uptake by kidney cells. He subjected his data to a compartmental analysis and isolated two influences. One was a very fast uptake of calcium which he tentatively ascribed to extracellular binding on the outer surface of the cells. The other slower influence appeared to be the entry of calcium into the cells (Fig. 6–2). It was therefore apparent that if the gradient across the plasma membrane of cells was so great, and if calcium could enter cells, then there must be some active process extruding calcium as fast as it entered.

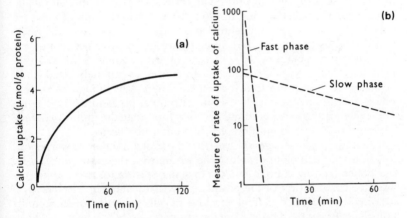

Fig. 6–2   (a) The uptake of calcium by kidney cells when placed in a solution containing 1.3 mmol/l calcium ions. (b) The curve obtained in (a) can be analysed to show that it consists of two components, the fast one of which is probably extracellular binding while the slow component represents calcium penetration into the cells. (Redrawn from BORLE, A. (1970), *J. gen. Physiol.*, **55**, 163–86.)

The general speculation about intracellular calcium was added to when R. V. TALMAGE began to obtain evidence that parathyroid hormone not only affected osteoclasts but also osteoblast cells. In both cases the hormone appeared to increase the amount of RNA (ribonucleic acid) and protein syntheses within the cells. Even more surprising, however, was the fact that the effects of parathyroid hormone could be mimicked by supplying calcium to the cells. It was suggested that perhaps parathyroid hormone produced its effects by permitting extra calcium to enter cells and increase the intracellular concentration.

It appeared, therefore, that calcium might be an important ion in controlling the activities of cells, and that all cells possessed a metabolic pump for maintaining low levels of intracellular calcium. If this pump was oriented on the opposite side of the cell to the sites of calcium entry then it would obviously have the effect of transporting calcium across the cell. Could such phenomena be important in initiating calcification?

Other aspects of bone physiology were also producing problems. It became difficult to explain the occurrence of certain trace elements which turned up again and again in the analyses of bone mineral. There was too much strontium in bone for it to be accounted for as a passive constituent. There was also too little magnesium and the bones of fish contained too much carbonate for it to be derived directly from the blood. The outstanding problem, however, was potassium. It was well known that potassium ions did not become bound to bone crystals and, in fact, crystals of calcium phosphate formed in potassium-rich media actually discriminated against this ion. But the water in bones contained massive amounts of potassium and this was not derived from contaminating tissues, for the cells accounted for only 20 per cent of the fluid and the remaining 80 per cent of extracellular fluid was still extremely rich in potassium. Furthermore, as animals aged they appeared to lose potassium from their bones even though there was relatively little change in either serum or cellular potassium (Table 6–1). The evidence began to accumulate, therefore, that the fluid in contact with the bone mineral must be very different from plasma.

The feelings of Talmage summarized those of a number of workers at this time. Something appeared to be wrong with the basic concepts in our understanding of bone and 'the final major stimulus to our thinking was a re-examination of the postulate originally made by Howard . . . in which he suggested that an envelope of cells separated the inorganic non-living portions of bone from the rest of the body' (TALMAGE, 1969).

Clearly, the ideas summarized in Fig. 6–1 no longer fit all the available evidence and the HOWARD concept that there is a cellular membrane around bone began to receive a great deal of attention.

Table 6–1 The potassium ion content of rat cortical bone of various ages. Valves are means ± standard deviations. (Data from CANAS, F., TEREPKA, A. R. and NEUMAN, W. F. (1969), *Amer. J. Physiol.*, **217**, 117–20.)

Weight of rats (g)	Number of rats used	Serum potassium (mmol/l)	Potassium in bone (mmol/l total water)
50	6	7.0 ± 0.3	303 ± 12
100	10	7.0 ± 0.3	135 ± 1
175	20	6.8 ± 0.3	130 ± 4
300	4	6.5 ± 0.3	129 ± 6

6.2   The bone-membrane hypothesis

As we have seen this theory was first proposed by HOWARD but it has been stated more directly by R. V. TALMAGE as consisting of five postulates. These are:

1. Bone contains two fluid compartments separated by a layer of cells (Fig. 6–3).

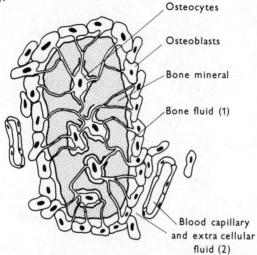

Osteocytes

Osteoblasts

Bone mineral

Bone fluid (1)

Blood capillary
and extra cellular
fluid (2)

Fig. 6–3   A diagrammatic representation of bone being covered by a cellular envelope. The bone fluid permeates the mineral and is in contact with osteocytes. It is separated by a layer of osteoblasts from the other extracellular fluids. (Modified after TALMAGE, R. V. (1969), *Clin. Orthop.,* **67**, 210–24.)

2. The inner fluid is associated with the mineralized tissue. The ionic calcium and phosphate concentrations of this fluid are controlled by the solubility product of the mineral and thus the concentrations of these ions are less than those in the extracellular fluid.
3. The outer fluid compartment can be thought of as equilibrating rapidly with the blood.
4. Since the calcium concentration on the two sides of the cell membrane are different, calcium is continually tending to enter the inner one and is continually being pumped out by the cells (Fig. 6–4).
5. Parathyroid and calcitonin hormones act by influencing the ability of these cells to move phosphate and calcium ions in and out of the fluid surrounding the bone mineral.

6.3   Implications of the theory

In 1971 NEUMAN, reviewing his work on the supersaturation of plasma with calcium and phosphate ions, was to write:

'In retrospect the whole issue now appears irrelevant. It should have been as obvious then as it is now. The mineral salts deposited in the skeleton are not in chemical equilibrium with the blood. It really does not matter what its solubility properties might be. The . . . data are clearly describing a case of disequilibrium . . . bone possesses a membrane or its functional equivalent that separates it from the circulation. . . ." (NEUMAN, W. F. and RAMP, W. K. 1971.)

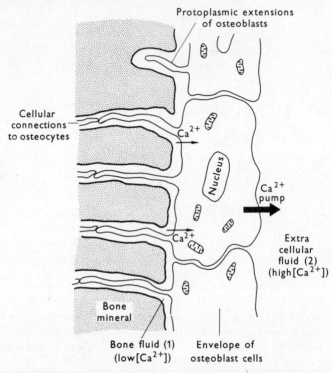

Fig. 6–4 The regulation of plasma calcium levels by the activity of the osteoblast envelope around bone. Bone fluid is in equilibrium with bone mineral but calcium which leaks into this fluid from the plasma is pumped out by the cells. (After TALMAGE, R. V. (1969), *Clin. Orthop.,* **67**, 210–24.)

This is a particularly harsh appraisal of his own excellent work which led on to the concepts of nucleation and crystal poisons. It is true, however, that if there is a functional membrane around bone which separates it from the blood system, then all the attempts to relate plasma ion concentrations to the solubility of bone are irrelevant. The membrane theory obviously has enormous implications here.

The anatomical evidence for a membrane around bone is not, however, entirely conclusive and it is certainly not a conspicuous structure or it would have been noted many years ago. It is true that the periosteal and endosteal surfaces are covered with cells and the fine spicules of trabecular bone are always covered with a cellular sheet, but there are not always continuous layers. In fact, the identification of the cells forming the membrane is difficult and 'all morphologists feel that there are "bare spots" in bone namely areas of apatite crystal not covered with cells' (TALMAGE, 1969). It is suggested that in those sites the crystals may be covered in pyrophosphate ions or other crystal poisons which convert the minerals into a relatively unreactive form.

Another implication of the membrane concept is that simple equilibria between plasma and bone mineral will not occur when radioisotopes are injected. Thus, the whole theoretical basis of the BAUER, CARLSSON and LINDQUIST analysis of bone accretion, resorption and exchange disappears if the specific activity of the plasma does not represent the specific activity of the fluid adjacent to the crystals.

Finally, the concept that there is a cellular layer between the bone mineral and the blood implies that it must be the activities of these cells which influence the formation of new bone. It is upon these cells that calcitonin and parathyroid hormone must act and this action must influence the movement of calcium and phosphate ions across these cells. These ideas are summarized in Fig. 6–5.

One is faced, therefore, with a remarkable situation. The simple

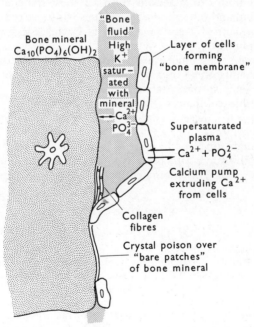

Fig. 6–5 A reinterpretation of the hypothesis shown in Fig. 6–1 in the light of the bone membrane concept.

anatomical suggestion that there may be a layer of cells around bone has led to a drastic revision of the significance of the measurements made on the solubility products of bone mineral in relation to plasma composition (Chapter 2), on the possible importance of crystal poisons (Chapter 3), on the mechanism of hormonal control (Chapter 4) and on the interpretation to be placed on kinetic experiments (Chapter 5). It must be stressed, however, that all the experimental work remains as accurate and repeatable as ever. The facts of science which form the basis of Chapters 2 to 5 remain unaffected. Only the hypothesis has changed from that summarized in Fig. 6–1 to that in Fig. 6–5—and hypotheses are simply suggestions made to help reasoning.

6.4 Conclusions and future work

It will be apparent from what has just been stated that biomineralization is a field of study which is still developing and thus difficult to summarize. One obviously needs, however, a basis for interpreting future work and discussing new concepts, and the following list is an attempt to provide that. It is based mainly upon bone physiology, but it is stated in a general form so as to be applicable to most examples of calcification.

1. Biomineralization will only occur in regions where the fluids tend towards conditions of supersaturation for those minerals, i.e. in sites where calcium and other ions accumulate so as to exceed the solubility produce constant of a particular type of crystal (e.g. hydroxyapatite, calcite, aragonite, etc.).

2. The process of biomineralization may be assisted by the presence of existing minerals or by organic matrices which act as sites for crystal overgrowth (epitaxy) or crystal nucleation.

3. Numerous substances will inhibit or poison these processes and such materials will therefore have to be excluded from the sites of actual mineral deposition.

4. The anions involved in mineral formation also act as buffers and exist in combination with protons at the pH of the body fluids (i.e. HCO_3^- and HPO_4^{2-}). Biomineralization involves displacing these protons, i.e.

$$Ca^{2+} + HCO_3^- \longrightarrow CaCO_3 + H^+$$

$$10Ca^{2+} + 6HPO_4^{2-} + 2H_2O \longrightarrow Ca_{10}(PO_4)_6(OH)_2 + 8H^+$$

Fig. 6–6 Cellular membranes involved in secreting various calcareous deposits: (a) the shell gland of the domestic fowl with 'uterine fluid' between the cells and eggshell; (b) the cellular endolymphatic sac extending from the inner ear of the amphibian tadpole and containing endolymph fluid and a calcareous deposit; (c) the extrapallial fluid between the mantle tissue and the shell of a bivalve mollusc.

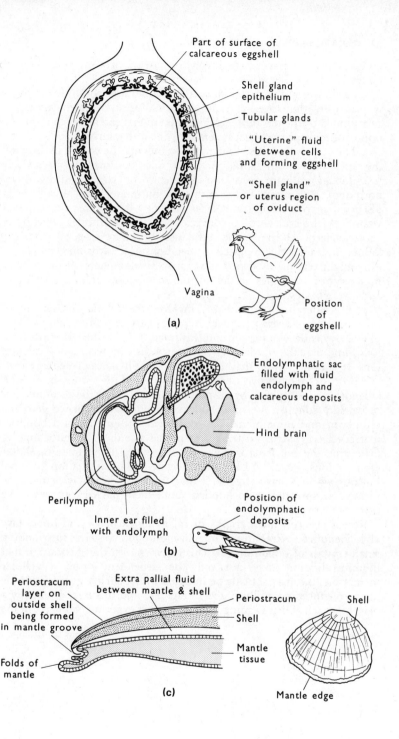

Part of surface of
calcareous eggshell

Shell gland
epithelium

Tubular glands

"Uterine" fluid
between cells
and forming eggshell

"Shell gland"
or uterus region
of oviduct

Vagina

(a)

Position
of
eggshell

Endolymphatic sac
filled with fluid
endolymph and
calcareous deposits

Hind brain

Perilymph

Inner ear filled
with endolymph

Position of
endolymphatic
deposits

(b)

Periostracum
layer on
outside shell
being formed
in mantle groove

Extra pallial fluid
between mantle & shell

Periostracum

Shell

Shell

Mantle
tissue

Folds of
mantle

(c)

Mantle edge

Calcification must therefore involve removing protons from sites of mineralization which would otherwise become acidic.

5. Factors 1–4 require special localized conditions within the body. It is probable, therefore, that most normal sites of calcification are surrounded by membranes (Fig. 6–6), and to that extent the concept of a bone membrane brings that system into line with many others.

6. The activities of these lining membranes may be critical in deciding the sites of biomineralization. They may be involved in actively transporting calcium ions and they may be controlled by many hormones. Calcitonin and parathyroid hormone have already been discussed in this respect and it has recently been demonstrated that vitamin D (cholecalciferol) is converted in the body into 1,25 dihydroxy cholecalciferol which is a powerful new hormone released from the kidney and affecting the calcium metabolism of birds and mammals. One might reasonably expect many new developments on the cellular influences of hormones on the calcium metabolism of both vertebrates and invertebrates.

7. Biomineralization probably involves the cellular movement of calcium ions or even complete mineral salts. A whole new field of physiology is developing around this interest. It has been known for a long time that the mitochondria within cells can accumulate calcium ions. It is now realized that this activity actually takes precedence over the process of oxidative phosphorylation and the synthesis of ATP (adenosine triphosphate) by the mitochondria. During the accumulation of calcium ions by the mitochondria protons are expelled into the cytoplasm and mineral may be deposited within the mitochondrial matrix (cf. 4). This is variously interpreted as either the mitochondria protecting the cell from damage by preventing a rise in intracellular calcium ions, or as a basic part of the biomineralization process. Various workers have suggested that bone mineral may actually be formed within the mitochondria and then passed out into the extracellular region.

Recent electron micrographs of calcifying cartilage and bone have also identified extracellular membrane-bound vesicles surrounding small crystals of bone mineral. This has increased the speculation that biomineralization may not only be dependent upon a cellular membrane, but may actually be initiated within such a structure. Some of these concepts are illustrated in Fig. 6–7 and this is undoubtedly a new approach which is going to attract much experimental work in the next few years.

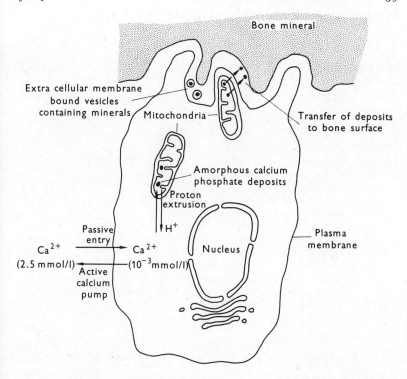

Fig. 6–7   Calcium enters cells down a concentration gradient but is continually being pumped out again by a metabolic pump in the plasma membrane. The mitochondria may be involved in maintaining the very low concentrations of calcium within the cytoplasm. In addition the mitochondria extrude protons and form mineralized deposits which may then be passed to the outside of the cell as part of the process of biomineralization. It has also been suggested that vesicles derived from cells may be a source of bone mineral.

References and Further Reading

The following papers provide the basis of the main experiments discussed in this book.

Key references

BAUER, G. H., CARLSSON, A. and LINDQUIST, B. (1955). Evaluation of accretion, resorption and exchange reactions in the skeleton. *Kungl. Fysiogr. Sallskap. Lund. Fiorhadl.,* **25**, 1–16

—— (1961). *Mineral Metabolism,* Vol. 1B. Edited by C. L. Comar, and F. Bronner, 609–76. London, Academic Press

COPP, D. H., CAMERON, E. C., CHENEY, B. A., DAVIDSON, A. G. F. and HENZE, E. G. (1962). Evidence for calcitonin—a new hormone from the parathyroid that lowers blood calcium. *Endocrinology,* **70**, 638–49

FLEISCH, H. and NEUMAN, W. F. (1961). Mechanisms of calcification: role of collagen, polyphosphates and phosphatase. *Am. J. Physiol.,* **200**, 1296–1300

TALMAGE, R. V. (1969). Calcium homeostasis—calcium transport—parathyroid action. *Clin. Orthop.,* **67**, 210–24

Further reading

BASSETT, C. A. L. (1968). Biological significance of piezoelectricity. *Calc. Tiss. Res.,* **1**, 252–72

—— (1965). Electrical effects in bone. *Sci. Amer.,* **213**, 18–25

BORLE, A. B. (1973). Calcium metabolism at the cellular level. *Fed. Proc.,* **32**, 1944–54

COPP, D. H. (1969). Endocrine control of calcium homeostasis. *J. Endocr.,* **43**, 137–61

LEHNINGER, A. L. (1970). Mitochondria and calcium ion transport. *Biochem. J.,* **119**, 129–38

NEUMAN, W. F. and NEUMAN, M. W. (1958). *The Chemical Dynamics of Bone Mineral.* Univ. Chicago Press

NEUMAN, W. F. and RAMP, W. K. (1971). The concept of a bone membrane: some implications. In *Cellular Mechanisms for Calcium Transfer and Homeostasis.* Edited by G. Nichols and R. H. Wasserman. London, Academic Press

SIMKISS, K. (1964). Phosphates as crystal poisons of calcification. *Biol. Rev.* **39**, 487–505

—— (1967). *Calcium in Reproductive Physiology.* London, Chapman and Hall

—— (1974). Calcium translocation by cells. *Endeavour,* **33**, 119–23

VAUGHAN, J. M. (1970). *The Physiology of Bone.* Oxford, Clarendon Press